Objective type questions and answers in

Veterinary Immunology

Dr. T.R. Kannaki, M.V.Sc.
Immunology Section,
I.V.R.I.

and

Dr. P.C. Verma, M.V.Sc., Ph.D.
Pr. Scientist,
I.V.R.I.

SCIENTIFIC PUBLISHERS (INDIA)

P.O. Box 91 JODHPUR

Published by:
Pawan Kumar
Scientific Publishers (India)
5-A, New Pali Road, P.O. Box 91
Jodhpur - 342 001 (Raj.)
Tel.: +91-291-2433323
Fax.: + 91-291-2512580
E-mail: info@scientificpub.com
www.scientificpub.com

ISBN: 978-81-7233-521-2

Laser typeset : Rajesh Ojha
Printed in India

Preface

Now a days students are in tough situation of tackling competitive environment. With the advances in educational system, the evaluation pattern has also been changed over time from traditional pattern to analytical pattern which needs deeper understanding and the ability to analyse.To cope up with system, students need more practice on their subject.

In an attempt to help the present situation we prepared the objective type questions and answers in Veterinary immunology covering essential aspects as well as wider areas. We prepared this book by keeping in mind about the competitive exams like ICAR-JRF, ICMR, CSIR-JRF and also semester exams of various Institutes.

We hope this book will be helpful for students as well as for teachers, we eagerly expect your comments and valuable suggestions to improve our work.

T.R. Kannaki
P.C. Verma

Contents

Chapter 1

Overview of immune system

Fill in the blanks

1. __________ and __________ demonstrated that dead organisms could also be used as vaccines.
2. An organism that can cause disease is said to be a ________, and their ability to cause disease is termed __________.
3. A technique called ________ was first followed by Lady mary wortley montagu.
4. __________ first coined the term vaccine, in honor of Jenner's work with cowpox inoculation.
5. Innate immunity comprises of four types of defensive barriers, namely, viz., __________, __________, __________ and__________ .
6. ________, a hydrolytic enzyme found in mucous secretions and in tears, is able to cleave the peptidoglycan layer of bacterial cell wall.
7. Adaptive immunity displays four characteristic attributes namely, __________, __________, __________ and __________.
8. The first disease that has been eradicated worldwide by the program of vaccination is __________.

Choose the best answer

9. Immune recognition is remarkable for its

(a) Sensitivity (b) Specificity
(c) Memory (d) Magnitude ( )

True or false

10. Opportunistic pathogens can cause disease only in immunosuppressed animals.
11. Innate immunity relies on the fact that invading microorganisms are chemically very different from normal body components.
12. Innate immune system possess memory.
13. The main distinction between the innate and acquired immune systems lies in their use of receptors to recognize foreign invaders.
14. Repeated injections of antigen lead indefinitely to greater and greater immune response.
15. Graft rejection is a specific immune response, and also possess memory.
16. Clonal selection theory is now accepted as the underlying paradigm of modern immunology.
17. Adaptive immunity is independent of innate immunity.
18. Memory B cells express the same membrane bound antibody as their parent B cells.
19. Invertebrates do not contain antigen-specific lymphocytes and do not produce immunoglobulin molecules or complement proteins
20. All normal immune responses wane with time after antigen stimulation, thus returning to its resting basal state.

Match

21. 1. Von Behring & kitasato – (a) Rabies vaccine

2. Elie Metchnikoff – (b) Small pox
3. Joseph resister – (c) Antitoxin
4. Edward jenner – (d) Phagocytes

22.

1. Side - chain theory – (a) Niels Jerne
2. Instruction theory – (b) Paul Ehrlich
3. Clonal selection theory – (c) Linus pauling

Answers

1. Daniel salmon and Theobald smith
2. pathogen, virulence
3. Variolation
4. Pasture
5. anatomic, physiologic, phagocytic and inflammatory
6. Lysozyme
7. specificity, diversity, memory and self/nonself recognition
8. small pox
9. b
10. True
11. True
12. False
13. True
14. False
15. True
16. True
17. False
18. True
19. True
20. True
21. 1. c, 2. d, 3. a, 4. b
22. 1. b, 2. c, 3. a

Chapter 2

Cells and organs of immune system

Fill in the blanks

1. A functional ______ gene is essential for the development of the lymphoid, erythroid and myeloid lineages.
2. Transcriptional factor _______ is required only for the development of cells of the lymphoid lineage.
3. bcl-2 and bcl-X_L genes encode protein products that _______ apoptosis.
4. Lymphocytes constitute _______% of the body's white blood cells and _______% of the cells in the lymph.
5. The ratio of $CD4^+$ and $CD8^+$ T cells is approximately _____ in normal human peripheral blood.
6. NK cells constitute ______% of lymphocytes in human peripheral blood.
7. Largest lymphatic vessel in body is _________.
8. M cells are located in so-called ________ sites small regions of a mucous membrane that lie over organized lymphoid follicles.
9. Langerhans cells contain characteristic granules called _______ granules.
10. ______ is an essential mineral for the development of T cells.
11. __________ are the martyrs of the immune system.

12. Innate resistance to Mycobacteria, Brucella, Leishmania and Salmonella is controlled by a gene ________Nramp coding for an ion transporter protein in macrophages.

13. Particles coated with antibody tend to be removed in _______ whereas particles coated with complement are preferentially removed in ________.

14. The success or failure of bacterial invasion is determined by the level of _______ is body fluids.

Choose the best answer

15. PALS of spleen is mainly populated by

    (a) B lymphocytes (b) T lymphocytes
    (c) Plasma cells (d) Memory cells ( )

16. Dendritic cells are found in all organs except

    (a) brain (b) eye
    (c) testes (d) all of the above ( )

17. Which of the following is zinc containing harmone ?

    (a) Thymosin (b) Thymopoietin
    (c) Thymulin (d) All of the above ( )

True or false

18. Apoptosis induce a local inflammatory response.

19. Only lymphocytes possess attributes of an adaptive immune response.

20. Activated lymphocytes are more susceptible to apoptosis than are naive lymphocytes or memory cells.

21. Stem cells express differentiation antigens.

22. CD45 is expressed uniquely by B-lineage cells.

23. CD40 and 40L interaction is essential for development of plasma cells and memory B cells.

24. TCR recognize free antigen.
25. Humans with Chediak-Higashi syndrome has increased incidence of lymphomas.
26. Beige mice lack NK cells.
27. NK1-T cell has some of the characteristic of both T cells and NK cells.
28. The rate of phagocytosis of an antigen is 4000 fold higher in the presence of specific antibody than its absence.
29. Both neutrophils and eosinophils are phagocytic whereas basophils are not.
30. Neutrophils exhibit larger respiratory burst than macrophages.
31. Neutrophils express lower levels of defensins than macrophages do.
32. Follicular dendritic cell arise in bone marrow and do not express closs II MHC molecules.
33. Nude mice fail to develop thymus.
34. Unlike lymph nodes, the spleen is not supplied by lymphatic vessels.
35. Most of the IELs express γδ TCR and exhibit limited diversity.
36. The pleuripotent stem cell is one of the most abundant cell types in the bone marrow.
37. Lymphoid follicles are present only in the spleen and lymph nodes.
38. Infection has no influence on the rate of hematopoiesis.
39. FDCs can process and present antigen to T lymphocytes.
40. All lymphoid cells have antigen-specific receptors on their membrane.

41. All vertebrates generate B lymphocytes in bone marrow.
42. All vertebrates produce B or T lymphocytes and most produce both.
43. Spleen contains germinal centres.
44. Lymph node but not spleen function is affected by a knockout of the Ikaros gene.
45. Lymphocytes are not found in jawless fishes.
46. Dendritic cells are 100 times more potent than macrophages and B cells.
47. Langerhans cells are specialized dendritic cells found in epidermis.
48. One dendritic cell may activate as many as 3000 T cells.
49. IL-12 producing dendritic cells are called DC1 cells whereas IL-4 producing dendritic cells are called DC2 cells.
50. TLR4 is expressed on myeloid dendritic cells and TLR9 is expressed on lymphoid dendritic cells.
51. Antigen processing by macrophages is inefficient.
52. Histiocytomas are common in the dog but rare in goats and cattle.
53. Bursin activates B cells but not T cells.
54. In contrast to naive T cells, memory T cells leave the blood stream through conventional blood vessels.
55. M2 cells generate nitric oxide.
56. TNF α is responsible for severe weight loss seen in animals with cancer.
57. Neutrophils constitute about 60-75% of blood leukocytes in most carnivores but only about 50% in horse and 20-30% in ruminants.

58. Granulysins are toxic peptides produced by cytotoxic T cells and NK cells.
59. Lysozyme is found in all body fluids except CSF, sweat and urine.
60. The three major types of sentinel cell receptors are called toll-like receptors.
61. Connective tissue and skin mast cells are rich in the molecules histamine and heparin, whereas intestinal mast cells contain chondroitin sulfate.
62. Intestinal mast cells remain at relatively constant levels whereas connective tissue mast cells can proliferate.
63. HEVs are present in the spleen.
64. Chemokines are chemoattractants for lymphocytes but not for other leukocytes.
65. Integrins are expressed on both leukocytes and endothelial cells.
66. Leukocyte extravasation involves multiple interactions between cell-adhesion molecules.
67. Mucin-like CAMs interact with selectins.
68. MAdCAM-1 is an endothelial adhesion molecule that binds to L-selectin and to several integrins.
69. Most circulating leukocytes express L-selectin, whereas E-selectin and P-selectin are expressed on vascular endothelial cells.
70. MAdCAM-1 has both Ig-like domains and mucin like domains.
71. Effector and memory cells express increased levels of certain cell adhesion molecules, such as LFA-1, that interact with ligands present on tertiary extra lymphoid tissue.

Match

72.

1. Histiocytes	–	(a) bone
2. Kupffer cells	–	(b) brain
3. Mesangial cells	–	(c) Kidney
4. Osteoclast	–	(d) connective tissue
5. Microglial cells	–	(e) Liver

Answers

1. GATA-2
2. Ikaros
3. Inhibit
4. 20-40%,99%
5. 2:1
6. 5-10%
7. thoracic duct
8. Inductive
9. Birbeck
10. Zinc
11. Neutrophils
12. Nramp
13. spleen, liver
14. iron
15. b
16. d
17. c
18. False
19. True
20. True
21. False
22. False
23. True
24. False
25. True
26. True
27. True
28. True
29. True
30. True
31. False
32. False
33. True
34. True
35. True
36. False
37. False
38. False
39. False
40. False
41. False
42. False
43. True
44. False
45. True
46. True

47. True
48. True
49. True
50. True
51. True
52. True
53. True
54. True
55. False
56. True
57. True
58. True
59. True
60. True
61. True
62. False
63. False
64. False
65. False
66. True
67. True
68. True
69. True
70. True
71. True
72. 1.d, 2.e, 3.c, 4.a, 5. b.

Chapter 3

Antigens

Fill in the blanks

1. ______________ is the ability to combine specifically with the final products of humoral or cell mediated immune responses.
2. Antigen administered intravenously is carried first to the __________ whereas antigen administered subcutaneously moves first to ______________.
3. Lymphocytes recognize discrete sites on the macromolecule called __________.
4. _________ is the portion of antigen interacting with MHC.
5. ___________ plot depicts the variability of amino acids in Ig molecule.
6. The overall strength of attachment of antigen with antibody molecule is known as _______________.
7. One epitope occurs for every __________ kD size protein.

Choose the best answer

8. Which of the following is potent immunogen ?

   (a) Proteins (b) Nucleic acids

   (c) Carbohydrates (d) Fat ( )

9. Lipids tend to be poor antigens because

(a) widely distributed (b) rapidly metabolised

(c) relative simplicity (d) Structural instability

(e) all of above ( )

10. Cross reaction occurs due to

(a) Coincidental similarity between unrelated molecules

(b) proteins evolutionarily related

(c) Structural similarities

(d) All of above ( )

11. Minimum molecular size for an antigen is

(a) 10 kD (b) 1000 D

(c) 100 D (d) 1000 kD ( )

12. Covalent association of heavy and light chains formed by disulfide bonds occurs in

(a) Ribosomes (b) Endoplasmic reticulum

(c) Golgi apparatus (d) None of the above ( )

True or false

13. Immunogenicity and antigenicity are related but distinct.

14. Although all molecules that have the property of immunogenicity also have the property of antigenicity, the reverse is not true.

15. Haptens possess immunogenicity.

16. Immunogenicity is an intrinsic property of an antigen.

17. The degree of immunogenicity of antigen depends on the degree of its foreignness.

18. APCs can degrade only proteins containing L-amino acids, polymers of D-amino acids cannot be processed.

19. B cell epitopes can contain sequential or nonsequential amino acids.
20. Epitopes recognized by T cells are often internal.
21. MBL and C-reactive protein (CRP) are soluble pattern receptors that bind to microbial surface and promote their opsonisation.
22. Most antigens induce a response from more than one clone.
23. A hapten can stimulate antibody formation but cannot combine with antibody molecules.
24. All antigens are also immunogens.
25. Antibodies can bind hydrophilic or hydrophobic compounds, but T-cell receptors can only bind peptide-MHC complexes.
26. Each MHC molecule binds a unique peptide.
27. T cell epitopes tend to be accessible amino acid residues that can combine with T-cell receptor.
28. Carriers are needed only if one wants to elicit a cell-mediated response.
29. B cell epitopes loose their immunogenicity when a protein antigen is denatured by heat.
30. Immunodominant T cell epitopes are determined in part by the MHC molecules expressed by an individual.
31. Multiple different epitopes may occur in the same antigen.

Match

32.

1. TLR 2	----	(a)	LPS
2. TLR 4	----	(b)	Peptidoglycan

3. TLR 5	-----	(c) Teichoic acid
4. TLR 9	-----	(d) Flagellin
5. TLR 6	-----	(e) CpG DNA

Define

33. Mimotope

Answers

1. Antigenicity
2. Spleen, local lymph nodes
3. Epitopes
4. Agretope
5. Kabat-Wu
6. avidity
7. 5 Kd
8. a
9. e
10. d
11. b
12. b
13. True
14. True
15. False
16. False
17. True
18. True
19. True
20. True
21. True
22. True
23. False
24. False
25. True
26. False
27. False
28. False
29. True
30. True
31. True
32. 1.b 2.a 3.d 4.e 5.c

Chapter 4

Antigen processing and presentation

Fill in the blanks

1. ________ and _________ are the two major pathway for processing and presentation of exogenous and endogenous antigens respectively.
2. $CD4^{+}$ and $CD8^{+}$ T cells can recognize antigen only when it is presented by a self MHC molecule. This is known as _________.
3. $CD4^{+}$ TH cells are _________ MHC restricted.
4. Self MHC restriction was demonstrated first by ________ and ________ in the year 1974.
5. Proteins targeted for degradation are attached with _______ and cleaved in multifunctional protease complex ____________.
6. Immunoproteasomes preferentially cleaves peptide bonds that follow _______ or ________ residues that bind to class I MHC molecules.
7. Molecular chaperones involved in MHC I assembly are _______ , _______ and ________.
8. The oligopeptides that bind to class II MHC molecule consists of _____ residues whereas MHC I molecule can bind to peptides of ______residues.
9. _________ is a Short fragment of invariant chain that remains bound with MHC II molecule after it is cleaved in endosomal compartment.

10. __________ is required to catalyze the exchange of CLIP with antigenic peptides.

11. ___________binds to HLA-DM and lessens the efficiency of peptide exchange reaction.

12. HLA-DO differs from HLA-DM is that it is expressed only by ______ and ________.

13. Molecular weight of proteasomes and immunoproteasome are _____ and ______kDa respectively.

14. Non protein antigens are presented by members of _______ family belongs to nonclassical class I molecules. CD1 genes can be induced by exposure to certain cytokines such as ______ or ______.

16. Preexisting antibodies greatly increase the efficiency of antigen processing by ________ and _________ cells.

17. Cytoplasm of dendritic cells contain characteristic granules called __________ granules.

18. __________ cells influence the development of skin allergies such as DTH and allergic contact dermatitis.

19. ________ cells are dendritic cells found in lymph that flows from tissues into lymph nodes, and represents transition between langerhan cells and interdigitating cells.

20. FDCs carry round beaded immune complexes on their filamentous processes known as ________ .

21. APC carries about _______ MHC II molecules that are capable of presenting peptides to T cells.

22. T cell can be activated by exposure to _________ number of peptide - MHC complexes.

Choose the best answer

23. Antigen processing and presentation can be prevented by,

(a) treating the APCs with paraformaldehyde

(b) Glutaraldehyde

(c) both of above

(d) None of above ( )

24. Professional antigen presenting cells are,

(a) Dendritic cells (b) Macrophages

(c) B cells (d) All of the above ( )

25. Most potent APC in processing naive antigen is

(a) B cells (b) Macrophages

(c) Dendritic cells (d) neutrophils ( )

26. Which cell express class II MHC molecules constitutively and co stimulatory molecules upon activation,

(a) Dendritic cells (b) B cells

(c) Macrophages (d) Fibroblast ( )

27. Cell that express class II MHC molecule and co stimulatory molecule upon activation only.

(a) Macrophages (b) Dendritic cell

(c) B cell (d) Target cell ( )

28. Assembly and loading of peptide in MHC I molecule takes place in

(a) Endoplasmic reticulum (b) Golgi vesicle

(c) Endosome (d) Plasma membrane ( )

29. Whether an antigenic peptide associates with class I or with class II is determined by,

(a) mode of entry into cell

(b) Either exogenous or endogenous

(c) Site of processing (d) All of above ( )

30. Macrophages internalize antigen by
    (a) Phagocytosis (b) Endocytosis
    (c) Both (d) None ( )

31. Endocytic pathway is inhibited by
    (a) Chloroquin/ lysomotropic agent
    (b) Leupeptin / protease inhibitors
    (c) Both
    (d) None ( )

32. The role of invariant chain (Ii, CD74) is,
    (a) Prevents binding of endogenous peptide with MHC II molecule
    (b) Involved in folding of class II α and β chain
    (c) Routing of MHC II to trans-golgi network.
    (d) All of above ( )

33. HLA-DO differs from MHC II genes in
    (a) Non classic and non polymorphic
    (b) Expression not induced by IFN-γ
    (c) α and β genes are not adjacent
    (d) all of above ( )

34. Which of the following cell is effective in presenting antigen to memory T cell and Th1 cell,
    (a) B cell (c) Dendritic cell
    (b) Macrophage (d) Fibroblast ( )

35. Macrophages are efficient phagocytic cells but not antigen presenting cell due to,
    (a) Phagocytosed antigen destroyed by lysosomal protease

(b) Need activation to express MHC II and co stimulatory molecule

(c) Both

(d) Neither a or b ( )

36. CD1 molecule can be recognized by

(a) Double positive T cell (b) Double negative T cell

(c) $\gamma\delta$ T cells (d) NK-T cells

(e) all of above ( )

37. Dendritic cells are the most effective APCs for initiating primary T cell responses due to,

(a) Located at the common sites of entry of microbes.

(b) Express receptors like TLR to catch microbe

(c) Migrate preferentially to T cell zone of LN.

(d) Constitutively express MHC II and co stimulatory molecules.

(e) all of above ( )

38. Peptides transported into the ER preferentially bind to class I, but not class II due to,

(a) Newly synthesized MHC I readily receive peptides.

(b) Ii chain blocks binding to MHC II

(c) both

(d) Neither of above ( )

True or false

39. Virtually any nucleated cell is able to function as a target cell presenting endogenous antigens to T_C cells.

40. APCs require 1-3 h to process and present antigen on its surface after exposure.

41. TAP molecules belong to the family of ATP binding casettes.
42. TAP1 and TAP2 genes are located outside the MHC region.
43. LMP genes and transporter genes are nonpolymorphic.
44. β2 microglobulin is covalently linked to MHC I.
45. Invariant chain is synthesized as trimers that associate with MHC II molecule.
46. Existence of two different antigen processing pathways was prooved by Morrison and Braciale.
47. Chloroquine inhibits endocytic pathway and cytosolic pathway is inhibited by emetine.
48. Proteasomes involved in antigen processing include two subunits namely LMP2 and LMP7.
49. LMP2, LMP7 and LMP10 levels can be increased by higher levels of IFNγ, T cell cytokine.
50. Molecular chaperones involved in MHC I assembly are located at ER.
51. B cells internalize antigen very effectively by receptor mediated endocytosis.
52. HLA-DM is not polymorphic and is not expressed at the cell membrane.
53. HLA-DO, and HLA-DM expression can be induced by IFN-γ.
54. Peptide bind strongly in compact form at plasma membrane at neutral pH that is difficult to replace by another peptide.
55. β2 microglobulin is coded by MHC genes.
56. There are five genes encoding human CD1 molecule located not within MHC but on chromosome 1.

57. All mammalian species studied have CD1 genes although the number varies.
58. Certain CD1 molecules are recognized by T cells in the absence of foreign antigens, and shows self restriction.
59. CD1 molecules are unable to process antigen in TAP deficient cells.
60. CD1 d molecules are recognized by NK cells.
61. CD1 molecule has general structural similarity to class I MHC and associate with β_2M.
62. UV inactivated influenza virus will be presented by Endocytic pathway.
63. Major source of non peptide antigen is Myocbacterium family.
64. CD1 pathway is different from classical MHC I pathway.
65. Macrophages can phagocytose organisms in the absence of antibody for opsonization.
66. Follicular dendritic cells are located in B cell area whereas interdigitating cells are lcoated in T cell area .
67. FDCs are present in all lymphoid tissues including thymus.
68. FDC are confined to the follicles in B cell areas.
69. Dendritic cells are poorly phagocytic but potent APCs when compared to macrophages.
70. One antigen presenting cell can present many epitopes to T cell simultaneously.
71. TAP-1 and TAP-2 heterodimer belongs to ATP binding cassette family.
72. Most T lymphocytes can recognize only peptides, so induced only by protein antigen.

73. Humoral immune responses are seen with protein and non protein antigens as B cell can recognize both.

74. T cells can distinguish peptides that differ even at single amino acid residue.

75. CD1 molecule presents non protein antigens to non MHC restricted $\gamma\delta$ T cells.

76. Vascular endothelial cells express MHC II and co stimulatory molecules constitutively in humans, but in mice it is inducible.

77. Dendritic cells after capturing antigen specifically migrate to T cell area of LN, as they express chemokine receptor CCR7.

78. Most abundant proteases of endosomes are cathepsins.

Match

79.

1. Syngenic ---- a. Identical except one allele
2. Congenic ----- b. Identical except one loci
3. Coisogenic ----- c. Identical at all loci

80. Match the pH of following cell oragnelles

1. Early endosome --- a. 4.5-5
2. Late endosome --- b. 6-6.5
3. Lysosome --- c. 5-6

81. Match

1. Emetine —— (a) increases pH of lysosome
2. Chloroquine —— (b) protein syntehsis inhibitor
3. leupeptin —— (c) protease inhibitor

82. Match the location of following dendritic cells

1. Langerhan cells —— a. cortex of LN
2. Interdigitating —— b. lymph
3. Follicular cells —— c. skin
4. Veiled cells —— d. paracortex of LN

83. Differentiate

Antigen presenting cell and Target cell

Antigen presenting cell	Target cell
(a) Display antigenic peptides associated with MHC II to $CD4^+$ TH cells	(a) Display peptides associated with class I MHC molecule to $CD8^+$ TC cells
(b) Only restricted population of cells can act as APCs	(b) Virtually all nucleated cells can act as target cells

84. Define

Self MHC restriction

Self MHC restriction is the attribute of T cells that limit their response to antigen associated with self MHC molecules on the membrane of antigen-presenting cells or target cells. In general, $CD4^+$ TH cells are class II MHC restricted and $CD8^+$ TC cells are class I MHC restricted.

85. Exogenous antigen and endogenous antigen

Exogenous antigen	**Endogenous antigen**
(a) Exogenous antigens are internalised by APCs	(a) Synthesised within altered self-cells

(b) Processed in endocytic pathway	(b) Processed in the cytosolic pathway
(c) Presented by MCH II molecules cells to CD4+ TH cells	(c) Presented by MHC I to CD8+ TC

86. **Give examples of non professional APCs**

(i) Fibroblasts
(ii) Glial cells
(iii) Pancreatic β cell
(iv) Thymic epithelial cells
(v) Thyroid epithelial cells
(vi) Vascular endothelial cells

87. Define cross priming / presentation

Answers

1. endocytic and cytosolic pathway
2. self MHC restriction
3. II class
4. Zinkernagel and P Doherty
5. Ubiquitin, proteasomes
6. basic or hydrophobic
7. calnexin, calreticulin and tapasin.
8. 13-18, 12-24
9. CLIP
10. HLA-DM
11. HLA-DO
12. B cells and thymus.
13. 700 and 1500 kDa
14. CD1
15. GM-CSF or IL-3.
16. dendritic cells and B cells.
17. Birbeck granules
18. Langerhan cells
19. Veiled cells
20. iccosomes
21. 2 x10^5
22. 200-300
23. c
24. d
25. c
26. b
27. a
28. a
29. d
30. c
31. c
32. d
33. d
34. a

35. c
36. e
37. e
38. c
39. True
40. True
41. True
42. False
43. False
44. False
45. True
46. True
47. True
48. True
49. True
50. True
51. True
52. True
53. True
54. True
55. False
56. True
57. True
58. True
59. False
60. True
61. True
62. True
63. True
64. True
65. True
66. True
67. False
68. True
69. True
70. True
71. True
72. True
73. True
74. True
75. True
76. True
77. True
78. True
79. 1.c, 2.b, 3.a
80. 1.b, 2.c, 3.a
81. 1.b, 2.a, 3.c
82. 1.c, 2.d, 3.a, 4.b

Chapter 5

Structure and function of antibodies

Fill in the blanks

1. First evidence of presence of antibodies in particular serum protein fraction was given by ________ and ________.
2. ________digestion of antibody molecule yield $F(ab)'_2$ fragment whereas ________ digestion yield 2 Fab fragment.
3. Hinge region is rich in ________ and ________ residues .
4. Large number of ________ residues in hinge region gives stability against proteolytic enzymes.
5. μ and ε chains lack ______region.
6. In humans there are ____ IgG subclasses.
7. The IgG subclasses of human differ in size of ______ region and the number and position of the interchain ________ bonds between the heavy chains.
8. ________ is a 70,000 MW-polypeptide comprising of five immunoglobulin like domains that bind to Fc region of IgA dimer.
9. Fc receptors for _____ antibodies are found in basophil and mast cells.
10. Mature B cell express _____ and _____class immunoglobulin on its membrane.

11. The sum of the individual idiotopes is called the _______ of the antibody.
12. Each individual antigenic determinant of the variable region is referred as _______.
13. _____ cell receptor is composed of mIg and disulfide linked heterodimers Ig-α/Igβ.
14. The term is ______ used to denote proteins whose corresponding genes derived from a common primordial gene encoding the basic domain structure.
15. Most members of the _________ super family can not bind antigen.
16. In 1975, _______ and _______ devised a method for preparing monoclonal antibody.
17. _________ comprises of tumor-specific monoclonal antibodies coupled to lethal toxins are potentially valuable therapeutic agents.
18. The toxins used in preparing immunotoxins include _____, _____ and _____ all of which inhibit protein synthesis.
19. ________ are produced by immunizing the mice with transition state analogue.
20. Catalytic antibodies, ________ have dual role as antibody and enzymes.
21. A saturable IgG protection _______ receptor regulates the half life of IgG.
22. ______ plot depicts the variability of amino acid residues in immunoglobulin molecule.
23. The average length of hyper variable region in Ig molecule is ___ residues.
24. Membrane bound antibody moleucles have extra hydrophobic transmembrane residues and basic intracytoplastic residues at ______.

25. The structure of Ig molecule was first elucidated by ______ and ________.

26. ________ are 100 kDa heavy chain dimers that lacks light chains found exclusively in camels. 27.Two signals necessary for class switching are from __________ and __________.

Choose the best answer

28. IgM class is found in which fraction of serum under electrophoresis ?

(a) α (c) γ

(b) β (d) Albumin

29. Heavy chain and light chain of antibody molecules are bound by,

(a) Disulfide bond (b) Hydrogen bond

(c) Hydrophobic bond (d) All of above

30. Disulfide linkage between two heavy chains of antibody moleucle is located in

(a) Fab region (b) Fc region

(c) Hinge region (d) Constant domain

31. CDRs involved in antigen binding is present in,

(a) Only in light chain (b) Only in heavy chain

(c) Heavy and light chain (d) Fc region

32. Role played by glycosylation of antibodies are,

(a) Increases the solubility

(b) Affects the rate of degradation

(c) Decreases the efficiency of interaction between ab and complement/Fc receptors

(d) All of above

33. Bence-Jones proteins are,

    (a) Light chains (b) heavy chains

    (c) Both heavy and light chain (d) None

34. Long hinge regi‹ n is present in,

    (a) IgM (b) IgD

    (c) IgG (d) IgA

35. Most abundant class in serum is,

    (a) IgM (b) IgG

    (c) IgA (d) IgD

36. Which subclass of IgG does not cross placenta ?

    (a) IgG3 (b) IgG1

    (c) IgG2 (d) IgG4

37. Which subclass of IgG is most effective complement activator ?

    (a) IgG3 (b) IgG1

    (c) IgG2 (d) IgG4

38. which subclass of IgG do not activate complement at all ?

    (a) IgG3 (b) IgG1

    (c) IgG2 (d) IgG4

39. Which subclass of IgG do not bind with protein A of *Staphylococcus aureus?*

    (a) IgG3 (b) IgG1

    (c) IgG2 (d) IgG4

40. Membrane bound IgM molecule is

    (a) Monomer (b) dimer

    (c) Pentamer (d) Tetramer

41. IgM secreted by plasma cell is a

(a) Monomer (b) dimer

(c) Pentamer (d) Tetramer

42. J chain is synthesized by

(a) B cell (b) Plasma cell

(c) Epithelial cell of mucous membrane

(d) None

43. Secretory component of IgA is synthesized by,

(a) B cell (b) Plasma cell

(c) Epithelial cell of mucous membrane

(d) None

44. Predominant Ig class in external secretions of primates is

(a) IgA (b) IgG

(c) IgM (d) IgD

45. Ig class synthesized in large quantity is

(a) IgA (b) IgG

(c) IgM (d) IgD

46. First Ig class produced in a primary response to an antigen is

(a) IgA (b) IgG

(c) IgM (d) IgD

47. Efficient Ig class in agglutination is

(a) IgM (b) IgG

(c) IgA (d) IgD

48. Efficient Ig class in precipitation is

(a) IgM (b) IgG

(c) IgA (d) IgD

49. Which component of IgA masks the sites from protease cleavage

    (a) J chain (b) Secretory component

    (c) Hinge region (d) Disulfide bond

50. The only Ig subclass that can act intracellularly,

    (a) IgG (b) IgA

    (c) IgM (d) IgE

51. When an antibody from one species is injected into another species, antibody response would be produced against,

    (a) Isotype (b) Allotype

    (c) Idiotype (d) None

52. Abzymes can be used in,

    (a) To cut peptide bonds at specific amino acid residue

    (b) To analyse sturcture and function of a protein

    (c) To block viral infectivity

    (d) To dissolve blood clots

    (e) All of above

53. Biological function of Fc region is / are,

    (a) Opsonisation (b) Complement activation

    (c) ADCC (d) Transcytosis

    (e) All of above

54. Naturally occurring antibodies against RBC's side chain in ABO blood group system belong to class,

    (a) IgG (b) IgM

    (c) IgA (d) IgE

55. Ig of choice for passive immunization against toxins and venoms is,

(a) IgG (b) IgM

(c) IgE (d) IgD

56. Mode of action of IgA in protection is

(a) Prevents the adherence of microbe

(b) Acts as opsonin

(c) Activates complement

(d) ADCC

57. The expression of Gm markers is

(a) Dominant (b) Recessive

(c) Co dominant (d) Partial dominant

58. Which of the following antigen binding site is highly variable ?

(a) CDR1 (b) CDR2

(c) CDR3 (d) Framework region

59. Isotypes of Ig differ in

(a) C region (b) V region

(c) Hinge region (d) Fab region

60. Long and many disulfide linkages are characteristics of which subclass of IgG in human ?

(a) IgG1 (b) IgG2

(c) IgG3 (d) IgG4

61. Two subclasses of IgE is found in

(a) Dog (b) Cat

(c) Cattle (d) Sheep

62. Two subclasses of IgA is found in

(a) Sheep (b) Chimpanzee

(c) Mouse (d) Human

(e) all

63. Which subclass of IgG predominates in horse used for tetanus immunoglobulin production ?

    (a) G1 (b) G2

    (c) G3 (d) G4

64. Cattle possess unique Fc receptor on macrophages and neutrophils that binds only to,

    (a) IgG1 (b) IgG2

    (c) IgM (d) IgA

True or false

65. Fc portion consists of both heavy and light chain.
66. Fragments of pepsin digestion of antibody molecule can still cross link antigen.
67. Pepsin cleaves the antibody molecule below the inter chain disulfide linkage whereas papain digests above the linkage.
68. Variable region is located in carboxy terminal and the constant region in amino terminal end of antibody molecule.
69. In humans, 60% of light chains are kappa where it is only 5% in mice.
70. There are no subtypes in K light chain.
71. There are three and 4 subtypes of λ light chain of mice and human respectively.
72. Each class of antibody can have either κ or λ light chain.
73. Each immunoglobulin fold consists of two antiparallel β pleated sheets connected by variable length of α loops.
74. C domain is slightly larger than V domain.
75. CDRs are located on variable length α loops.

76. In general, more residues in the heavy chain CDRs appear to contact antigen than in the light chain CDRs.
77. CH1 and CL domains enhances the flexibility of Fab arms.
78. Heavy chains in IgE and IgM contain four constant domains and no hinge region.
79. CH2/CH2 domains in IgE and IgM occupy the same position as hinge region of other classes.
80. The antigenic specificity of all the membrane antibody molecules expressed by single B cell is identical.
81. The class of all membrane bound antibody molecule on single B cell is identical.
82. The capacity to undergo transplacental transport depends upon properties of the variable region of antibody molecule.
83. Less IgM than IgG is required to neutralize viral infectivity.
84. IgG is more efficient than IgM in activating complement.
85. IgM is found in high concentration in the intracellular tissue fluids.
86. Everyday, a human secretes 5 to 15 g of IgA into mucous secretions.
87. Poly Ig receptor is a suicidal receptor.
88. Poly Ig receptor interacts with the J chain of both polymeric IgA and IgM antibodies.
89. Each isotype is encoded by a separate constant region gene.
90. All members of a species carry the same constant region genes.

91. Within a species, each individual will express all isotypes in the serum.
92. Different species express different isotypes.
93. Antibodies to allotypic determinants do not arise from blood transfusion.
94. Isotypic determinants are located at variable region of both heavy and light chain.
95. Idotope are variable region sequences, may be the actual antigen-binding site or located outside.
96. γ chain allotypes are referred as Gm markers.
97. Empirical formula for an antibody is H_2L_2 or H_2K_2 / $H_2 \lambda_2$.
98. Igβ chain has longer cytolasmic tail than Ig α chain.
99. Fc receptors have been discovered only for few Ig classes.
100. All the FcRs belong to immunoglobulin super family.
101. All myeloma protein molecules derived from a single myeloma clone have the same idiotype and allotype.
102. A rabbit immunized with human IgG3 will produce antibodies that react with all subclasses of IgG in humans.
103. Monomeric IgA can undergo transcytosis.
104. Polymeric IgM and IgA dimers undergo transcytosis.
105. IgG developed much more recently during evolution than IgM.
106. IgG diffuses more readily to intercellular fluid.
107. Half life of IgG increases at high concentration.
108. Hinge region is absent in IgM and IgE.
109. J chain is present in IgM and IgA.

110. Efficient Ig class in complement activation is IgG.
111. Free IgM molecules appear as star shaped, after binding with antigen they appear as crab.
112. IgA activates complement.
113. IgA can't act as opsonin.
114. IgD has long hinge region connected by disulfide linkage.
115. IgD is reported in pigs, rabbits and dometic mammals.
116. IgD is more prone to proteases.
117. IgA is predominant isotype in cow's milk.
118. In humans, IgG subtypes are numbered based upon serum concentration.
119. C region of immunoglobulin mediates most of the biological function.
120. C region participates in antigen binding.
121. C regions of light chains participate in effector functions.
122. Different isotypes and subtypes of antibodies perform different effector functions.
123. An antibody molecule has either two k light chains or two λ light chains, but never one of each.
124. K and λ light chains differ in their C region.
125. There are functional differences in k containing and λ containing antibodies.
126. N glycosylation of antibody molecules occurs at endoplasmic reticulum and its modification occurs at golgi complex.
127. Bovine IgG2 agglutinates antigenic particles, whereas IgG1 does not.
128. Rabbits have as many as 13 IgA subclasses.

129. All the heavy chain constant region genes are located together on one chromosome.

130. IgG3 of horse does not activate complement and produce characteristic flocculation.

131. IgG2 levels in bovine is highly heritable.

132. All the great apes, with the exception of the orungutan, have two IgA subclasses.

133. Rabbits have only one IgG heavy IGHG chain gene despite having IGHA genes.

134. IgG1 of bovine has faster electrophoretic mobility than IgG2.

135. All heavy chain constant region genes are generally arranged in the order of 5'-Cμ - Cδ - Cγ - Cε - Cα - 3' .

136. Match

1. μ ----- (a) IgD
2. γ ----- (b) IgE
3. α ----- (c) IgA
4. δ ----- (d) IgM
5. ε ------ (e) IgG

137. **Match** the length of cytoplasmic tail with Ig class.

1. IgM, IgD – (a) 28
2. IgA – (b) 14
3. IgG, IgE – (c) 3

138. Match

1.IgE --- a. Less abundant isotype in serum
2.IgM --- b. Efficient toxin neutralization.
3.IgD --- c. Binds to Fc receptors on mast cells.
4.IgG --- d. Present on surface of immature B cell

139. Match the half lives with Ig class

1.IgM	–	(a) 6 days
2.IgG	–	(b) 3 days
3.IgA	–	(c) 10 days
4.IgD	–	(d) 21 days
5.IgE	–	(e) 2 days

140. Match the IgG subclasses with the species

1. Horse	–	a. G1, G2a, G2b, G3, G4
2. Cattle	–	b. G1, G2, G3, G4
3. Mouse	–	c. G1, G2a, G2b, G3
4. Dog	–	d. G1, G2, Ge
5. Pig	–	e. G1, G2, G3, G4, G5, G6

141. Match the sedimentation coefficient with Ig class :

1. IgM	–	(a) 11s
2. IgA dimer	–	(b) 8s
3. IgE	–	(c) 19s
4. IgG	–	(d) 7s
5. IgD	–	(e) 7s

142. Match the moleuclar weight with Ig class

1. IgM	–	(a) 180 kDa
2. IgA	–	(b) 180 kDa
3. IgE	–	(c) 200 kDa
4. IgG	–	(d) 900 kDa
5. IgD	–	(e) 360 kDa

143. Match the carbohydrate content with Ig class

1. IgD	–	(a) 8%
2. IgM	–	(b) 12%

3. IgA – (c) 13%
4. IgG – (d) 3%

144. Match the on and off rate of the following antigen binding molecules.

1. Ig – (a) slow on rate, very slow off rate
2. TCR – (b) Slow on rate, slow off rate
3. MHC – (c) Rapid on rate, variable off rate

145. Match the affinity of antigen binding of the following molecules

1. Ig – (a) 10^{-6} M
2. TCR – (b) $10^{-5} - 10^{-7}$ M
3. MHC – (c) $10^{-7} - 10^{-11}$ M.

Answers

1. Tiselius, Kabat
2. Pepsin, papain
3. proline, cysteine
4. proline
5. Hinge
6. 4
7. Hinge, disulfide
8. Secretory component
9. IgE
10. IgM, IgD
11. Idiotype
12. idiotype
13. B
14. super family
15. immunoglobulin
16. Georges kohler, Cesar milstein
17. Immunotoxins
18. ricin, shigella toxin and diptheria toxin
19. Abzymes
20. Abzymes
21. Bambrell
22. Kabat-wu
23. 10
24. C terminal
25. Porter and Edelman
26. Nanobodies
27. CD40 : CD40L and cytokines
28. b
29. d
30. c
31. c

32. d
33. a
34. b
35. b
36. a
37. a
38. d
39. a
40. a
41. c
42. b
43. c
44. a
45. a
46. c
47. a
48. b
49. b
50. b
51. a
52. e
53. e
54. b
55. a
56. a
57. c
58. c
59. a
60. c
61. a
62. e
63. b
64. b
65. False
66. True
67. True
68. False
69. True
70. True
71. True
72. True
73. True
74. False
75. True
76. True
77. True
78. True
79. True
80. True
81. False
82. True
83. True
84. False
85. False
86. True
87. True
88. True
89. True
90. True
91. True
92. True
93. False
94. False
95. True
96. True
97. True

98. False
99. False
100. True
101. True
102. True
103. False
104. True
105. True
106. True
107. False
108. True
109. True
110. False
111. True
112. False
113. True
114. False
115. False
116. True
117. False
118. True
119. True
120. False
121. False
122. True
123. True
124. True
125. False
126. True
127. True
128. True
129. True
130. True
131. True
132. True
133. True
134. True
135. True
136. 1.d, 2.e, 3.c, 4.a, 5.b
137. 1.c, 2.b, 3.a
138. 1.c, 2.d, 3.a, 4.b
139. 1.c, 2.d, 3.a, 4.b, 5.e
140. 1.e, 2.d, 3.c, 4.b, 5.a
141. 1.c, 2.a, 3.b, 4.d, 5.e
142. 1.d, 2.e, 3.c,4.a, 5.b
143. 1.c, 2.b, 3.a, 4.d
144. 1.c, 2.b, 3.a
145. 1.c, 2.b, 3.a

Chapter 6

Major histocompatability complex

Fill in the blanks

1. Expression of non classical _______ MHC I molecules on cytotrophoblasts at the feto-maternal interface prevents fetal rejection.

2. Two chains of class II MHC molecules are encoded by __________, ________ regions in mice and by __________, ________, __________ regions in humans.

3. Class III products include complement components ____ ,____ ,_____and inflammatory cytokines TNF and HSPs.

4. Any one individual expresses ____ different MHC I moelcules and upto _____different class II molecules.

5. The recombination frequency of MHC loci is very low, only ______%.

6. Bare lymphocyte syndrome is caused by defect in transcriptional factor _____ and _______.

7. Mutation rate of MHC genes is ______/ gene/generation.

8. α_3 domain of I MHC binds to_______whereas β_2 region of class II MHC molecule binds to______in T cell.

9. Extraordinary polymorphism of MHC molecules has been generated by _______and not by ________.

10. ________serve the major source of genetic material for gene conversion.

11. MHC II products are constitutively expressed on all resting T cells of dogs, cats and horses but not in _______.

12. In ______ resting T cells can function as antigen presenting cells.

13. Class I MHC molecule and β_2 M are classified as members of __________ superfamily.

Choose the best answer

14. MHC participates in the development of

(a) humoral immunity (c) self and nonself recognition

(b) CMI (d) all of above

15. Characteristics of MHC genes are,

(a) Highly polymorphic (c) Inherited as haplotype

(b) Codominant (d) all of above

16. Which of the following statement is true regarding F1 hybrid of two inbred mouse strain differing at MHC loci.

(a) F1 hybrid is histocompatible with both strain

(b) F1 hybrid accept graft from either parental strain.

(c) Inbred parental strain can accept graft from F1 mice.

(d) a and b true.

17. When father and mother have different haplotypes, which of the following statement is true, about siblings,

(a) 1/4 chance that siblings are histocompatible

(b) None of the offspring will be histocompatible with parents

(c) Both are true

(d) Neither true

18. Which peptide bind to class I molecule with 100 to 1000 fold higher affinity?

(a) Octomer (b) Nonamer

(c) Hexamer (d) Decamer

19. In which of the following species MHC II molecules are normally expressed on renal vascular endothelium and glomeruli.

(a) Dog (b) Human, pig

(c) Cat (d) Bovine

20. In cattle, which of MHC II gene loci is absent ?

(a) DP (b) DQ

(c) DR (d) A

21. In equine ELA complex is linked to which of the the blood group system?

(a) A (b) B

(c) C (d) D

22. In swine SLA complex is linked to which of the the blood group system?

(a) J and C (b) B

(c) C (d) D

23. DP genes are absent in

(a) Cattle (b) Sheep

(c) Both (d) Goat

24. HLA-G is found only in,

(a) Human (b) Gorillas

(c) Chimpanzee (d) Rhesus monkey

25. HLA-C is found in

(a) Human (b) Gorillas

(c) Chimpanzee (d) All of above

26. Class II molecules can be detected in

(a) Pro B cell (b) Pre B cell

(c) Immature B cell (d) Mature B cell

27. Avian MHC genes are distinguished from mammalian MHC in that

(a) Chicken MHC genes are organized in two independent clusters.

(b) Class III genes of complement not yet reported.

(c) MHC haplotype differ in the individual I and II genes expressed

(d) all of the above

True or false

28. NK cells express receptors for MHC I antigens.

29. Major histocompatability complex is located on chromosome 6 in humans and 17 in mice.

30. Class III MHC genes code for secreted proteins that involve in both immune and non-immune function.

31. Class I MHC molecules are encoded by K&D regions in mice and by A, B and C loci in humans.

32. β_2 M contain a transmembrane region and is noncovalently bound to class I molecule.

33. Peptide binding groove of MHC I is formed by α_1 and α_2 domains.

34. Peptide binding by class I and II molecules exhibit fine specificity.

35. The peptide-binding cleft in class I molecules is blocked at both ends, whereas the cleft is open in class II molecules.
36. In normal healthy cells class I molecules display self peptides.
37. IL-4 increases expression of class II by resting B cells.
38. Expression of class II by B cells is upregulated by IFN-γ.
39. In autoimmune diseases MHC plays an important but not exclusive role.
40. No single MHC allele has been found to be present at high frequency.
41. MHC genes are present only in vertebrates.
42. All cells express MHC I molecule.
43. The majority of the peptides displayed by class I and class II MHC molecules on cells are derived from self-proteins.
44. Human RBCs are non nucleated and do not express any MHC molecule.
45. β_2-micro globulin is invariant among all class I molecules.
46. MHC molecules of an individual do not discriminate between foreign peptides and self peptides.
47. β_2 micro globulin is encoded by a gene on chromosome 15 in humans and 2 in mice.
48. Human but not mouse, T cell express class II molecules after activation.
49. Class Ib genes are highly polymorphic.
50. MHC I molecule is not found on mouse RBC.
51. The variable region of MHC molecule is located almost exclusively in the walls of the groove.

52. FcRn is a class Ib MHC molecule that does not have an obvious antigen binding groove and its gene is not located in MHC.

53. In cattle most MHC II molecules are expressed only on B cells and activated T cells.

54. Match

1. BoLA- Awl6 — (a) Resistance to BLV
2. B^2, B^6, B^{14}, B^{21} — (b) Marek's resistance
3. B^1, B^3, B^{15} — (c) Resistance to mastitis
4. BoLA-Aw7 — (d) Marek's susceptible

55.

1. RMAs cell line — (a) defective β_2 M.
2. Daudi tumor cells — (b) defective TAP genes

56.

1. Human — (a) ELA
2. Dog — (b) SLA
3. Cattle — (c) B
4. Horse — (d) HLA
5. Swine — (e) DLA
6. Mouse — (f) H-2
7. Chicken — (g) BoLA

57.

1. Non classical MHC II in mice — (a) DM, DO
2. Nonclassical MHC II in human — (b). Oα, Oβ, Mα, Mβ

58.

1. Ankylosing spondylitis – (a) DR2
2. IDDM – (b) DR4/DR3
3. Narcolepsy – (c) B 27
4. Rheumatoid arthritis – (d) DR3
5. SLE – (e) DR4

59. **Match** the level of expression of class I MHC by the following cells

1. High level — (a) Neurons, sperms
2. Low level — (b) Liver, muscle, fibroblast
3. Absent — (c) Lymphocytes

60.

1. Highly polymorphic – (a) Mouse, human
2. Less polymorphic – (b) Whale, elephant, seal, cat, mouse
3. Monomorphic – (c) Cheetah.

61. Explain why ?

The binding of a peptide and an MHC molecule is referred as promiscous.

Peptide binding by MHC moelcule does not exhibit fine specificity. Instead, a given MHC molecule can bind numerous different peptides and some peptides can bind to several different MHC molecules. Because of this broad specificity, binding of a peptide and an MHC molecule is referred as promiscous.

62. Explain the theories proposed to account for the variability in immune response among different haplotypes ?

(a) Determinant selection model : Different class II MHC molecules differ in their ability to bind processed antigen

(b) Holes-in-the-repertoire model : T cells bearing receptors that recognize foreign antigens closely resembling self-antigens may be eliminated during thymic processing.

63. Give examples of viruses that down regulates MHC I molecule

(i) CMV (iii) Adenovirus 12

(ii) HBV

64. Define : Linkage disequilibrium

It is the difference between the frequency observed for a particular combination of alleles and that expected from the frequencies of the individual alleles.

65. Differentiate peptide binding cleft of I and II MHC

MHC I	MHC II
a. Closed at both ends	Open cleft
b. Formed by α_1 & α_2 domains	formed by α_1 and $\beta_1$domains
c. Binds to 8-10 peptide	13-18 residues.

66. Differentiate

TCR/BCR	MHC
(a) Generation of TCR/BCR is dynamic, changing over time within an individual	(a) MHC molecules expressed by an individual are fixed in the genes and do not change over time
(b) Diversity generated by gene rearrangement and somatic mutation	(b) Diversity arise from polymorphism and multiple alleles

Answers

1. HLA-G
2. IA, IE and DP, DQ, DR
3. C4, C2, BF
4. 6, 12
5. 0.5
6. CII TA , RFA
7. 10^{-3}
8. CD8, CD4
9. gene conversion, point mutation
10. Pseudo genes
11. Mouse
12. pigs
13. immunoglobulin
14. d
15. d
16. d
17. a
18. b
19. b
20. a
21. a
22. a
23. c
24. a
25. d
26. d
27. d
28. True
29. True
30. True
31. True
32. False
33. True
34. False
35. True
36. True
37. True
38. False
39. True
40. True
41. True
42. False
43. True
44. True
45. True
46. True
47. True
48. True
49. False
50. False
51. True
52. True
53. True
54. 1.c, 2.b 3.d, 4.a
55. 1.b, 2.a
56. 1.d, 2.e, 3.g, 4.a, 5.b, 6.f, 7.c
57. 1.b, 2.a
58. 1.c, 2.b, 3.a, 4.e, 5.d
59. 1.c, 2.b, 3.a

Chapter 7

Immunoglobulin gene rearrangement

Fill in the blanks

1. Gene rearrangement in B cell was first proved by __________ and __________.
2. J gene segment codes for _____amino acids in the light chain of Ig molecule.
3. Each RSS contains a conserved __________ heptamer and a conserved _______ rich nonamer.
4. David schatzy, Marjorie Oettinger and Baltimore identified ____________ genes in 1990.
5. Joining of gene segements during rearrangement occurs in two ways, namely _________ joining and ________ joining.
6. Somatic mutation is mediated by a B cell enzyme called _______________.

Choose the best answer

7. 'D' gene segment of Ig heavy chain has which type of RSS on both sides?

   (a) One turn (b) two turn

   (c) both (d) None

8. Allelic exclusion is essential in lymphocytes for

   (a) To make them monospecific

(b) To make them multispecific

(c) To make them nonspecific

(d) None

9. Joining of which sequences in Ig gene rearrangement is imprecise ?

(a) Coding sequence

(b) Signal sequence

(c) Coding-signal sequence

(d) Signal-coding sequence

10. Which of the following process does not occur exclusively in CDR3 of Ig molecule?

(a) Junctional flexibility (b) P addition

(c) N addition (d) Somatic hypermutation

11. P addition during gene rearrangement generate ________ type of sequences

(a) Palindromic (b) Repetitive

(c) Non coded (d) None

12. Which of following enzyme is responsible for 'N' addition during gene rearrangement ?

(a) RAG -1 (b) RAG -2

(c) TdT (d) DSBR enzyme

13. N addition in antibody molecule occurs only in

(a) heavy chain (b) light chain

(c) both (d) hinge region

14. Normally, somatic hypermutation occurs only within

(a) Bone marrow (b) Paracortex

(c) Germinal centre (d) All of the above

15. Somatic hypermutation occurs at the frequency of

    (a) 10^{-3} / bp/gen (b) 10^{-6} / bp/ gen

    (c) 10^{-9} / bp / gen (d) 10^{-10} / bp/gen

16. Most of the mutation in somatic hypermutation are,

    (a) Substitution (b) deletion

    (c) insertion (d) Frameshift

17. Membrane bound and secreted form of antibody molecules differ in

    (a) N termini (b) C termini

    (c) Fab region (d) Variable region

18. Simultaneous expression of IgM and IgD on mature B cell is due to,

    (a) absence of switch region between Cμ and Cδ

    (b) differential RNA processing

    (c) Cμ and Cδ are located close and sequentially

    (d) All of above

19. Rate of transcription of immunoglobulin genes in unrearranged B cell is lower due to,

    (a) Weak binding of RNA polymerase II with promoters

    (b) Enhancers are located far from promoters

    (c) Both

    (d) None

20. Immunoglobulin gene rearrangement in T cell is inhibited by,

    (a) Absence of RAG genes (b) Absence of TdT

    (c) Pu1 binding site (d) DSBR enzyme

21. In immunotoxin, Fc region is intentionally destroyed to avoid

(a) Killing of non specific cells by binding via FcR

(b) Complement activation

(c) ADCC (d) Opsonisation

22. Somatic mutation of Ig genes accounts for,

(a) Allelic exclusion (c) affinity maturation

(b) Class switching (d) All of the above

23. The mechanism that permits Ig to be synthesized in either a membrane bound or secreted form is

(a) Allelic exclusion (b) Co dominant expression

(c) Class switching (d) Differential RNA processing

24. Which one of the following class switching can occur ?

(a) IgM to IgD (c) IgE to IgE

(b) IgA to IgG (d) IgM to IgA

25. The frequency of somatic mutation in Ig genes is greatest during,

1. Differentiation of pre B cells into mature B cells

2. Diffentiation of pre T cells into mature T cells

3. Generation of memory B cells

4. All of above

26. How many chances a B cell can take to generate a functional light chain gene ?

(a) 1 (b) 2

(c) 3 (d) 4

27. A B cell becomes immunocompetent following
    (a) rearrangement of variable region of heavy chain genes
    (b) rearrangement of variable region of both heavy chain and light chain genes.
    (c) Class switching
    (d) During affinity maturation

28. The major bonds formed between antigen and its receptor are
    (a) hydrophobic (b) Hydrogen
    (c) Ionic (d) Vander waals

29. Binding of a receptor to its antigen is mediated by multiple
    (a) Covalent bonds (b) Noncovalent bonds
    (c) both (d) None

30. Somatic mutation occurs in the following isotypes except,
    (a) IgG (b) IgA
    (c) IgM (d) IgE

31. The main process of generating Ig diversity in chicken is
    (a) gene conversion (b) Multiple 'V' genes
    (c) Somatic mutation (d) Combinational diversity

32. In which species, gut flora or antigenic stimulation is not absolutely necessary for 'v' gene diversification
    (a) Rabbit (b) Human
    (c) Mouse (d) Sheep

33. Antigen receptor diversity is mediated by
    (a) gene recombination (b) Somatic mutation
    (c) gene conversion (d) all of above

True or false

34. Pig B cells do undergo receptor editing.
35. Ig genes can't be transcribed and translated into complete chains until they are rearranged into functional genes.
36. Individual B cell is antigenically committed to multiple epitopes.
37. Lymphocyte cell lineage does not retain an intact copy of genomic DNA.
38. Genomic rearrangement occurs in all type of cells.
39. Different classes of antibody can be expressed with identical variable region sequences.
40. Light chain gene family contains V, J and C gene segments.
41. Heavy chain gene family contains V, D, J and C gene segments.
42. There are no subtypes in Κ light chain of immunoglobulin molecule.
43. RAG genes and TdT are the only lymphoid specific gene products that are involved in gene rearrangement.
44. One turn RSS have 23 bp spacer whereas two turn RSS have 12 bp spacer.
45. Vκ signal sequence has one-turn spacer and Jκ signal sequence has two-turn spacer. In λ light chain the order is reversed.
46. 'N' addition requires template.

47. Only less than 1/9 of the early stage pre-B cell progress to maturity and leave bone marrow as mature B cells.
48. B cell expresses rearranged heavy chain genes and light chain from both the chromosomes.
49. All V_H, D or V_L gene segments are used at same frequency during gene rearrangement.
50. Switch region is absent between Cμ and Cδ.
51. Oct 2 a transcriptional factor found only in B cells.
52. Heteroconjugates are hybrids having monospecificity.
53. Separate exons encode the transmembrane portion of each membrane immunoglobulin.
54. The antigen receptors on T and B cells have evolved to deal with specific microbial antigens.
55. The strength of non covalent bonds increases as the distance between antigen and its receptor increase.
56. On average, one mutation occurs each time a B cell divides.
57. Somatic mutation does not begin until after B cells have switched from IgM to either IgG or IgA.
58. Chicken has only a single functional V gene at its heavy and light chain gene loci.
59. Species that undertake gene conversion also show limited somatic mutation although the reverse is not true.
60. Appendix is the primary lymphoid oragn in rabbit.
61. Immunoglobulin diversity mechanisms are same in all species.
62. The diversity of the TCR V region is generated by gene recombination and combinatorial association in all species.

63. Immature T cell use α chain, as they mature, they switch to use δ chains.

64. Neither somatic mutation nor gene conversion occurs in TCR genes.

65. Looping out and deletion account for more than 75% of TCR rearrangements.

66. N addition and base deletion are much more extensive in immunoglobulin genes than in TCR genes.

67. In sheep γ/δ heterodimer occurs in at least five forms.

68. Match the target of commercially available mAb

1. Orthoclone OKT3	---	(a) CD200
2. Zenapax	---	(b) CD 52
3. Campath	---	(c) CD3
4. Rituxan	---	(d) CD25
5. Herceptin	---	(e) HER 2R

69. Define : Humanized antibody

* Engineering an antibody to contain promoter, leader and variable sequences from a mouse antibody gene and the constant region exons from a human antibody gene. The antibody encoded by such a recombinant gene is a mouse-human chimera, known as humanized antibody.

Answers

1. S. Tonegawa and Hozumi
2. 13
3. Palindromic, AT
4. recombination activating
5. inversional ,deletional
6. cytosine deaminase
7. a
8. a
9. a
10. d
11. a
12. c
13. a
14. c
15. a
16. a

17. b
18. d
19. c
20. c
21. a
22. c
23. d
24. d
25. d
26. d
27. b
28. a
29. b
30. c
31. a
32. d
33. d
34. False
35. True
36. False
37. True
38. False
39. True
40. True
41. True
42. True
43. True
44. False
45. True
46. False
47. True
48. False
49. False
50. True
51. True
52. False
53. True
54. False
55. False
56. True
57. True
58. True
59. True
60. True
61. False
62. True
63. False
64. True
65. True
66. False
67. True
68. 1.c,2.d,3.b,4.a,5.e

Chapter 8

Lymphocytes

Fill in the blanks

1. The pattern of cell surface molecules expressed on a cell is called as ________________.

2. B cell accounts for ____________% of circulating lymphocyte.

3. CD4/CD8 ratio of peripheral blood lymphocyte population in horse is ___________.

4. CD4/CD8 ratio of peripheral blood of most animals ranges from ________.

5. The peptide-binding cleft in _______ is blocked at both ends, whereas the cleft is open in ____________.

6. Naive T cell express ________ levels of CD45R and α-selectin and _________ levels of CD44.

7. Memory T cells express _______ levels of CD45R and L-selectin and _________ levels of CD44.

8. In adult cattle about __________% of ciruclating T cells are γ/δ positive and remainders are α/β positive.

9. T cell receptor is associated on the membrane with a signal-transuding complex _______ whose function is similar to that of Igα-Igβ complex of BCR.

10. The cytoplasmic tails of the CD3 chains contain a motif called _______

11. 50% of lymphocytes in the small bowel mucosa of chicken and mouse are $\gamma\delta$ T cells. They are known as ________________ .

12. ______ is a signal transducing molecule that is noncovalently associated with the cytoplasmic tails of CD4 and CD8.

13. CD45 is originally called as ________________ .

14. The principal ligand for CD2 in humans is __________.

15. P selectin found in secretory granules of endothelial cells are called ______________ bodies.

Choose the best answer

16. T and B lymphocytes can be differentiated by
    (a) size (b) staining property
    (c) Surface molecule (d) None

17. Cells involved in acquired immune response is
    (a) NK cell (b) Macrophage
    (c) Neutrophil (d) Lymphocytes

18. Which mitogen stimulates both B and T cell ?
    (a) Con A (b) PHA
    (c) Pokeweed (d) LPS

19. PHA and Con A are specific mitogens for stimulating
    (a) T cell (b) B cell
    (c) both (d) None

20. Which of the following statement about Thy-1 is true ?
    (a) In mice it is found on both thymocytes and blood T cells
    (b) In rat it is found on thymocytes but not in blood T cells

(c) In humans it is found on neither

(d) All are ture

21. Which peptide binds to class I molecule with 100 to 1000 fold higher affinity?

(a) Octomer (b) Nonamer

(c) Hexamer (d) decamer

22. Anchor residues for MHC I are located at

(a) 2nd position (b) 3rd

(c) 9th position (d) All of above

23. Predominant circulating T cells in ruminants is

(a) γ/δ^+, $WC1^+$, $CD4^-$, $CD8^-$

(b) α/β^+, $WC1^-$, $CD4^+$, $CD8^-$

(c) γ/δ^+, $WC1^+$, $CD8^+$, $CD4^-$

(d) α/β^+, $WC1^-$, $CD4^-$, $CD8^+$

24. Predominant circulating T cells in human and mice is

(a) γ/δ^+, $WC1^+$, $CD4^-$, $CD8^-$

(b) α/β^+, $WC1^-$, $CD4^+$, $CD8^-$

(c) γ/δ^+, $WC1^+$, $CD8^+$, $CD4^-$

(d) α/β^+, $WC1^-$, $CD4^-$, $CD8^+$

25. Which of the following statement about flow cytometry is true ?

(a) Scatter of light beam in a forward direction measures cell's size

(b) Scatter of light to side, measures surface roughness

(c) Only a true

(d) Both a and b are true

26. TCR resembles,

(a) Antibody molecule (b) Fab

(c) Fc (d) F(ab2)'

27. Transmembrane domains of TCR contain following type of amino acid residues ?

(a) Positively charged (b) Negatively charged

(c) Neutral (d) None

28. 60% γδ T cells are

(a) $CD4^+$ cells (b) $CD8^+$ cells

(c) Double positive cells

(d) Double negative cells

29. Productive rearrangement of α chain gene in TCR expression deletes

(a) δ gene (b) γ gene

(c) β gene (d) None

30. Which chains of TCR receptor are similar to light chains of BCR ?

(a) α and γ (b) β and δ

(c) α and β (d) γ and δ

31. Which chains of TCR receptor are similar to heavy chains of BCR

(a) α and γ (b) β and δ

(c) α and β (d) γ and δ

32. "D" segment coding for variable region of TCR is absent in

(a) α chain (b) γ chain

(c) both a & b (d) β chain

33. Self reactive T cells are eliminated by

(a) Negative selection in thymus

(b) Absence of somatic mutation

(c) both

(d) None

34. T cell receptor diversity is more than Ig diversity due to,

(a) More V gene segments in TCR DNA

(b) Alternative joining of D gene segment

(c) N addition occurs in all chains

(d) Both b and c

35. Which process is absent in TCR gene rearrangement

(a) N addition (b) P addition

(c) Junctional flexibility

(d) Somatic hyper mutation

36. Exceptions to allelic exclusion are most often seen in which TCR chain genes?

(a) α chain (b) β chain

(c) γ chain (d) δ chain

37. Which of the following two chains of CD3 complex are endoded by same gene ?

(a) $\gamma\varepsilon$ (b) $\delta\varepsilon$

(c) $\xi\eta$ (d) None

38. Cytoplasmic tail of CD4 contains ______ residues that can be phosphorylated

(a) Tyrosine (b) Serine

(c) Threonine (d) None

39. Which region of TCR chain is the binding site for super antigens ?

(a) $V\beta$ domain (b) $V\alpha$ domain

(c) $V\gamma$ domain (d) $V\delta$ domain

40. In TCR molecule interchain disulfide linkage is located at

(a) V region (b) C region

(c) Between V and C domain

(d) Below the C region

41. Longest intracytoplasmic tail is present in which of the polypeptide of CD3 compelx ?

(a) ε (b) δ

(c) ζ (d) γ chain

42. CD8 is a

(a) αβ heterodimer (b) Monomer

(c) Tetramer (d) None

43. ζ chain of CD3 complex is also present in

(a) B cell (b) NK cell

(c) Macrophages (d) Monocyte

44. γδ expressing T cells are abundant in

(a) Skin of mouse (b) Bowel mucosa of chicken

(c) Bowel mucosa of mice (d) All

45. Which of the following is not true about the accessory molecules of T cell

(a) Enhances the strength of adhesion between T cells and APCs

(b) Responsible for homing of T cells in tissues

(c) They are polymorhic

(d) Useful cell surface markers for identification

46. Which of the following statement about T cell co receptors CD4/CD8 is wrong?

(a) Promotes adhesion of T cells with APC

(b) Participate in early signal transduction of T cell activation

(c) Provides MHC restriction

(d) Provides antigen specificity

47. T cell coreceptors play a major role in,

(a) adhesion (b) signaling

(c) homing (d) antigen recognition

48. In humans, CD28 is expressed mainly on,

(a) $CD4^+$ T cell (b) $CD8^+$ T cell

(c) Double positive T cells

(d) Double negative T cell

49. CTLA 4 upon stimulation,

(a) activates T cell

(b) Inhibits T cell activation

(c) No role in T cell activation

(d) None

50. CTLA 4 is expressed on

(a) Naive T cells (b) recently activated T cells

(c) both (d) none

51. Which of the following molecule has longest cytoplasmic tail ?

(a) CD45 (b) CD44

(c) CD3 (d) CD4

52. Cytoplasmic domain of CD45 has intrinsic, ________ activity

(a) tyrosine kinase (b) tyrosine phosphatase

(c) Protein kinase (d) None

True or false

53. Antibodies are simply soluble BCRs.
54. CD3 is found on all T cells.
55. 65% of human T cells are $CD4^+$ and 30% are $CD8^+$ cells.
56. FcR for IgM and IgD have not yet been identified.
57. CD32 - B1 is found on B cells which regulates its function.
58. Integrins are heterodimeric proteins classified according to their α chain.
59. ICAM-1 is normally expressed only on dendritic cells and B cells.
60. Unlike ICAM-1, ICAM-2 is expressed on unstimulated endothelial cells and is not increased during inflammation.
61. CD2 is only found on T cell.
62. CD58 is the ligand for CD2.
63. Thy-1 is absent on the surface of astrocytes, epidermal cells and fibroblasts.
64. In cattle $WC1^+$ T lymphocytes are found in high numbers in skin and mucous membrane as well as in hemal nodes and thymus.
65. Any one individual expresses 6 different MHC I molecules and up to 12 different class II molecules.
66. Peptide binding by class I and II molecules does not exhibit the fine specificity.
67. MHC includes genes with similar, but not identical structure and function and said to be polygenic.
68. MHC spans 2000 kb of mouse DNA and some 4000 kb of human DNA.

69. Non classical MHC I genes in mice are H-2 or, T and M.
70. In humans the non classical class I genes include the HLA-E, F, G, HFE, J X and MIC.
71. In human DR region, there are three or four functions β chain genes but just one α chain gene.
72. Presence of linked class III gene cluster is conserved in all species.
73. The affinities of CD4 and CD8 for MHC molecules are very high.
74. Young calves have less γ/δ T cell proportion than adult cattle.
75. Unlike humans, bovine CD4 is not found on macrophages.
76. Double negative T cells may reach 80% in newborn calves.
77. In pigs, SWC1 is expressed on resting T cells, monocytes and granulocytes but not on B cells.
78. Only pigs have two subpopulation of γ/δ T cells.
79. All pig $CD4^+$ cells are α/β cells.
80. In dogs CD4 is expressed on monocytes but not on macrophages.
81. BCG is a B cell mitogen.
82. T cell receptors are specific not for antigen alone but also for MHC molecules.
83. The concept that specificity for both MHC and antigen residues in a single receptor was proved by the experiments of kappler and Marrack.
84. There is an additional hyper variability region in α chain of TCR. 85. TCR chain contains a short cytoplasmic tail of 5-12 residues at 'c' terminal.

86. γδ T cells are MHC restricted.
87. TCR V gene germ line repertoire is more for γδ T cells.
88. The genes that encode the αβ and γδ TCRs are expressed only in cells of T cell lineage.
89. The δ gene segments encoding for TCR are located between the V_α and J_α segments.
90. αβ TCR receptor can be co expressed with γδ receptor.
91. α and β chains of TCR are not linked to each other.
92. The germline DNA encoding for TCR constant region is much simpler than BCR constant genes.
93. TCR α chain DNA has only single C gene segment whereas the β chain DNA has two C gene segment.
94. TCR gene rearrangements do not follow the one-turn/two-turn joining rule.
95. Same enzymes are involved in the rearrangements of B cells and T cells.
96. Allelic exclusion is less stringent for TCR α genes than for β chain genes.
97. TCR variable domains have three hyper variable regions which are equivalent to CDRs of Ig molecule.
98. Location of one-turn and two-turn RSSs in TCR β chain and δ chain DNA is similar to that of Ig heavy chain DNA.
99. One D_δ gene can join with another D_δ gene in TCR gene rearrangements.
100. N addition occurs only in the Ig-heavy chain genes.
101. N addition occurs only in heavy chains of TCR molecule.
102. TCR DNA has far fewer V gene segments than Ig DNA.

103. CDR3 of the TCR has greater diversity than that seen in immunoglobulin.

104. TCR genes undergo extensive somatic mutation.

105. αβ heterodimer expression is not essential for membrane expression of αβ and δγ TCR.

106. CD3 is a complex of five invariant polypeptide chains that associate to form three dimers.

107. 90% of CD3 complexes incorporate the ξη heterodimer.

108. γ, δ and ε chains of CD3 are members of immunoglobulin super family.

109. Transmembrane region of all the CD3 polypeptide chains contain positively charged residues.

110. ξ and η chains of CD3 contains three copies of ITAM whereas other chains have only one copy.

111. CD4 is a 55 kDa monomeric membrane glycoprotein containing four extracellular domains.

112. Monoclonal antibody specific for CD4 will co precipitate the T cell receptor along with CD4.

113. Subtractive hybridization can be used to enrich for mRNA that is present in one cell type but absent in another cell type within the same species.

114. Clonotypic monoclonal antibody was used to isolate the T cell receptor.

115. TCR is bivalent and has two antigen binding sites.

116. Mechanisms for generation of diversity of TCR are identical to that of Igs.

117. The T cell uses the same set of V, D and J gene segments as the B cell but uses different C gene segments.

118. TCR is a clonally distributed receptor.

119. CD3 molecule is covalently linked to TCR complex.

120. TCR is produced both in membrane bound form and secreted form.
121. BCR is produced only in membrane bound form.
122. Isotype switching is found in TCR chains.
123. Only very few residues of peptide are responsible for the specificity of T cell antigen recognition.
124. The affinity of TCR for peptide-MHC complexes is much lower than that of most antibodies.
125. Virtually all αβ TCR expressing cells are MHC restricted.
126. Antibodies against TCR αβ heterodimer coprecipitation the CD3 polypeptides.
127. An ITAM motif contains two copies of the sequence W-X-X-L, separated by six to eight residues.
128. During maturation of T cells, TCR genes are expressed before the CD3 genes.
129. Only 10% of γδ T cells are $CD3^+$.
130. In mouse skin, most of itnraepidermal T cells express αβ receptor.
131. In humans, 90% of intraepithelial lymphocytes express γδ receptor.
132. γδ T cells require antigen processing and presentation before they are being recognized.
133. Accessory molecules of T cells are non polymorphic and invariant.
134. CD4 is also present in mononuclear phagocytes and some dendritic cells.
135. Some $CD4^+$ T cells, that are MHC class II restricted can act as CTLs in humans.
136. Cytoplasmic tail of CD8 is longer than CD4.

137. Knockout mice lacking CD4 cells do not contain MHC I restricted T cells.

138. T cell corecepors play a minor role in T cell APC adhesion.

139. The best defined co stimulator for T cells are B7-1 and B7-2 expressed on professional APCs.

140. CD28 is expressed on more than 90% of $CD4^+$ T cells and on 50% of $CD8^+$ T cells in humans.

141. CTLA 4 is expressed on naive T cells.

142. Naive human T cells express an isoform of CD45 RA whereas memory T cells express CD45RO isoform.

143. CD45 mediated dephosphorylation may allow LCK to become active.

144. Naive T cells express high levels of CD44.

145. CD44 is essential for retention of T cells in extra vascular tissues.

146. Activated T cells express ligand for the death receptor fas.

147. Virtually naive T cells express no E and P selectin ligands.

148. TH1 cells express significantly more selectin ligands than do Th2 cells.

Match

149.

1. L-selectin	– (a) Platelets
2. E-selectin	– (b) Endothelial cells
3. P selectin	– (c) Leukocyte

150.

1.T cell in LN – (a) follicular area
2. B cell in LN – (b) PALS
3. T cell is spleen – (c) Paracortex
4. B cell in spleen – (d) Cortex

151.

1. FC γRI, CD 64 – (a) B cell, macrophage
2. FC γRII, CD 32 – (b) Macrophages
3. FC γ RIII, CD 16 – (c) NK cells

152. Match the source of following mitogens

1. Con A – (a) Pokeweed plant
2. PHA – (b) Gram negative bacteria
3. Pokeweed – (c) Jack bean
4. LPS – (d) Red kidney bean

153.

1. CD11a/CD18 – (a) C3b
2. CD11b/CD18 – (b) ICAM-1
3. CD11c/CD18 – (c) fibrinogen

154.

1. Non classical MHC II in mice – a. DM, DO
2. Nonclassical MHC II is human – b. Oα, Oβ, Mα, Mβ

155. **Match** the level of expression of class I MHC by the following cells.

1. HIgh level – a, Liver, muscle, fibroblast
2. Low level – b. neurons, sperms
3. Absent – c. lymphocytes

156. Explain why ?

- The binding of a peptide and an MHC molecule is referred as promiscous.

Peptide binding by MHC molecules does not exhibit fine specificity. Instead, a given MHC molecule can bind numerous different peptides and some peptides can bind to several different MHC molecules. Because of this broad specificity, binding of a peptide and an MHC molecule is referred as 'promiscuous'.

157. Differentiate

	TCR/BCR	MHC
*	Generation of TCR/BCR is dynamic, changing over time within an individual	MHC molecules expressed by an individual are fixed in the genes and donot change over time
*	Diversity generated by gene rearrangement and somatic mutation	Diversity arise from polymorphism and multiple alleles

Define

158. Linkage disequilibrium

It is the difference between the frequency observed for a particular combination of alleles and that expected from the frequencies of the individual alleles.

159. Immunological synapse

The TCR and accessory molecules in the T cell plasma membrane more coordinately with their ligands in the APC membrane to form a transient supramolecular structure that has been called the immunological synapse.

Answers

1. Immunophenotype
2. 10-50%
3. 4.75
4. 1.4-1.9
5. class I molecules ,class II molecules
6. high, low
7. low, high
8. 10-15%
9. CD3
10. ITAM
11. intraepithelial lymphocytes
12. LCK
13. Leucocyte common antigen
14. LFA-3
15. Weibel-Palade
16. c
17. d
18. c
19. a
20. d
21. b
22. d
23. a
24. b
25. d
26. a
27. a
28. d
29. a
30. a
31. b
32. c
33. c
34. d
35. d
36. a
37. c
38. b
39. a
40. d
41. c
42. a
43. b
44. d
45. c
46. d
47. b
48. a
49. b
50. b
51. a
52. b
53. True
54. True
55. True
56. True
57. True
58. False
59. True
60. True
61. True
62. True
63. False
64. True
65. True
66. True
67. True

68. True
69. True
70. True
71. True
72. True
73. False
74. False
75. True
76. True
77. True
78. True
79. True
80. False
81. False
82. True
83. True
84. False
85. True
86. False
87. False
88. True
89. True
90. False
91. False
92. True
93. True
94. False
95. True
96. True
97. True
98. False
99. True
100. True
101. False
102. True
103. True
104. False
105. False
106. True
107. False
108. True
109. False
110. True
111. True
112. False
113. True
114. True
115. False
116. False
117. False
118. True
119. False
120. False
121. False
122. False
123. True
124. True
125. True
126. True
127. True
128. False
129. True
130. False
131. False
132. False
133. True
134. True
135. True
136. False
137. False

138. True
139. True
140. True
141. False
142. True
143. True
144. False
145. True
146. True
147. True
148. True
149. 1.c, 2.b, 3.a
150. 1.c, 2.d, 3.b, 4.a
151. 1.b, 2.a, 3.c
152. 1.c, 2.d, 3.c
153. 1.b, 2.c, 3.a
154. 1.b, 2.a
155. 1.c, 2.a, 3.b

Chapter 9

T and B cell maturation, activation and Differentiation

Fill in the blanks

1. ________ cytokine secreted by stromal cells is essential for B cell development.
2. Pre B cell receptor comprises of ________ and ________ known as surrogate light chain.
3. B-1 cells compose about _____% of the total B cell population.
4. Activation of T_H cells results in secretion of ________ cytokine and expression of its receptor, leading to proliferation and differentiation.
5. The rate of antibody synthesis by plasma cells is _______ per second.
6. Initial activation of naive B cells induced by thymus dependent antigens occurs within the ___________ of lymph nodes.
7. ___________ are rapidly dividing B cells located in the dark zone of germinal centres.
8. Centrocytes expressing high affinity mIg interact with antigen captured by ___________ in the light zone.
9. Generation of ___________ cells in the light zone of germinal centres is induced by interaction of centrocytes with IL-1 and CD3.

10. ______________ which occurs in proliferating centroblasts is critical for affinity maturation.

Choose the best answer

11. Immature B cells express which of the following isotype ?

    (a) IgM (b) IgD

    (c) IgE (d) IgG

True or false

12. B cell activation and maturation in the periphery require antigen.
13. Before birth, yolk sac, fetal liver and bone marrow are the major sites for B cell maturation.
14. TdT enzyme is active in pre B cell stage.
15. N addition are usually found in V_L-J_L joints.
16. Each pre B cell undergoes multiple cell divisions producing 32 to 64 descendants.
17. B-1 population responds poorly to protein antigens but much better to carbohydrate one.
18. Most thymus independent-1 antigens are polyclonal B cell activators.
19. TI -2 antigens activate both mature and immature B cells.
20. Only one Igα/Igβ heterodimer associates with single mIg molecule to form the recpetor complex.
21. TCR, and BCR itself has protein tyrosine kinase activity.
22. CD22 constitutively associated with B cell receptor in resting B cells, delivers a negative signal.

23. B cell coreceptor is composed of CD19, CR2 and TAPA-1.
24. B cell is able to present antigen to T_H cells at antigen concentration that are 100 to 10,000 times lower than required by macrophages or dendritic cells.
25. T_H cells and B cells, each recognizing different epitopes on the same antigen.
26. Plasma cells lack detectable membrane bound immunoglobulin.
27. BASAP is expressed only by B-lineage cells and influences all the cell stages during B cell maturation.
28. Heavy chain V_H-D_H-J_H rearrangement begins in the pre B cell stage.
29. In order to develop into immature B cells, pre B cells must interact directly with bone-marrow stromal cells.
30. Most centrocytes die by apoptosis in the light zone.
31. Immunization with a hapten-carrier conjugate results in production of antibodies to both hapten and carrier epitopes.
32. If mice are immunized with HRBCs and then are immunized a day later with SRBCs, the antibody response to the SRBCs will be much higher than that achieved in control mice immunized only with SRBCs.
33. The rearrangement of α chain genes of TCR does not begin until the double positive thymocytes stop proliferating.
34. The MHC haplotype of the thymus in which T cells develop determines their MHC restriction.
35. Positive selection ensures self tolerance and negative selection ensures MHC restriction.

36. CD28 is expressed by both resting and activated T cells but CTLA-4 is virtually undetectable on resting cells.
37. The suppression by regulatory T cells are antigen non specific.
38. LCK and ZAP-70 are protein kinases.
39. Calcineurin, a protein phosphatase is involved in generating the active form of the transcription factor NFAT.
40. Knockout mice lacking class I MHC molecules fail to produce thymocytes bearing CD8.
41. PIP_2 is split by a phospholipase to yield DAG and IP3.

Define

42. Original antigenic sin

Answer

1. IL-7
2. V pre B and λ 5
3. 5%
4. IL-
5. 1000
6. paracortex
7. Centroblast
8. follicular dendritic cells
9. memory
10. Somatic hypermutation
11. a
12. True
13. True
14. False
15. False
16. True
17. True
18. True
19. False
20. True
21. False
22. True
23. True
24. True
25. True
26. True
27. True
28. False
29. False
30. True
31. True
32. False

33. True
34. True
35. False
36. True
37. False
38. True
39. True
40. True
41. True

Chapter 10

Cell mediated effector responses

Fill in the blanks

1. The effectors of the humoral branch are mainly mediated by __________.
2. Th1 effector cells remain bound to _______ that display peptide-class II MHC complexes; Th2 effector cells remain bound to ______ that display peptide-class II MHC complexes.
3. Membrane bound molecules on effector T cells include ___________ and ______.
4. The proliferation and differentiation of both antigen activated TH1 cells and CTL-Ps depends upon the cytokine ______.
5. CTLs kill the target cells by two mechanisms namely _______ and _____ mediated pathways.
6. Granzyme B can also bind to ________ receptor on target cell surface and internalized to induce apoptosis.
7. CTLs use granzymes and Fas ligand to initiate _______ cascade in their target to induce apoptosis.
8. NK cells constitute about _____% of circulating lymphocyte population.
9. In ________ syndrome NK cells are lacking.

10. Almost all NK cells express _______, a receptor for the Fc region of IgG.

11. NK cells, unlike T cells, do not undergo ______ development.

12. Two major groups of inhibitory receptors found on NK cells are, _________ and _______.

13. The amount of _____ on the surface serves as indicator of the overall level of class I MHC biosynthesis in the cells.

14. The ______ is an *in vitro* system for assaying T_H-cell proliferation in a CMI response.

15. ________ is an *in vitro* assay of effector cytotoxic function.

16. _________ provides an *in vivo* system for studying cell mediated cytotoxicity.

17. Antigen non specific cells are made specific by a process called _____.

18. A spleen index of _____or greater is considered to be indicative of a positive GVH reaction.

19. For the activation of macrophages, the cytokines essential are _____and _________.

20. Nitric oxide derived from activated macrophages increases the expression of ______receptor on T cells.

21. Extrinsic apoptotic pathway is triggered by _____.

22. Extrinsic apoptotic pathway leads to the formation of ______ complex whereas intrinsic apoptotic pathway leads to the formation of _________.

23. Memory T cells are ______ positive cells and express high levels of _____ cytokine receptor.

24. Division of memory T cell requires ______cytokine and is inhibited by ________ cytokine.

25. The magnitude of clonal expansion of $CD4^+$ T cells is considerably less than that of $CD8^+$ T cells.

26. Signature cytokine of T_H1 subset is __________, whereas it is __________ for TH2 subset.

27. __________ is an antibacterial peptide found in the granules of both cytotoxic T cells and NK cells.

28. Effector T cells that migrate preferentially to the skin express a carbohydrate ligand called __________ that binds to E-selectin.

29. T cells that migrate to the intestine express an integrin called ______________.

Choose the best answer

30. Following are nonspecific cells except one involved in cell mediated immune response ?

    (a) NK cells (b) Macrophages

    (c) eosinophils (d) CTLs

31. In Di-George syndrome, immunity against _____ lacks

    (a) Intracellular pathogen (b) extra cellular pathogen

    (c) None (d) both

32. In persons with CMI deficiency which type of vaccine should be avoided ?

    (a) Killed vaccine (b) live attenuated

    (c) DNA vaccine (d) Recombinant vaccine

33. Generation of CTLs from CTL-precursors need

    (a) TLR – MHC I-peptide trimolecular complex signal

    (b) Co stimulatory signal

    (c) IL-2 signal

    (d) all of the above

34. After clearance of antigen, antigen specific TH1 cells and CTLs undergo programmed cell death by

    (a) Decline in the level of IL-2

    (b) Lack of antigen for stimulation

    (c) both of the above

    (d) None

35. Antigen specific activated CTLs can kill

    (a) Only one target cell (b) few target cells

    (c) Many (d) None

36. Firm adherence of CTLs with target cell for transient period is facilitated by

    (a) TCR-MHC I complex (b) Co stimulatory molecules

    (c) LFA-1 (d) all

37. Perforins of CTL has sequence homology with

    (a) C3 (b) C5

    (c) C9 (d) C8

38. Granzymes are,

    (a) Proteases (b) DNases

    (c) RNases (d) None

39. *Lpr* mice has mutated

    (a) Fas gene (b) Fas ligand gene

    (c) FADD (d) None

40. FADD is associated with

    (a) Procaspase 8 (b) Procaspase 3

    (c) Procaspase 9 (d) None

41. NK cells are nonspecific cells invovled in

    (a) Innate immunity (b) Adoptive immunity

    (c) Both (d) None

42. IFNγ derived from NK cells has inhibitory effects on

(a) TH1 cells (b) TH2 cells

(c) Macrophages (d) dendritic cells

43. NK cells constitutively express which subunit of IL-2 receptor,

(a) α (b) β

(c) γ (d) None

44. First line of defence against viral infection and intracellular bacteria is mediated by,

(a) Neutrophils (b) NK cells

(c) CTLs (d) Macrophages

45. Activation, proliferation and differentiation of CTL-P cells into functional CTLs requires

(a) 3 days (b) 5 days

(c) 7 days (d) 14 days

46. NK cells recognize the target cells by,

(a) MHC restriction (b) lack of MHC molecule

(c) Presence of specific peptide

(d) None

47. HLA-E bind to peptides derived from,

(a) HLA-A (b) HLA-B

(c) HLA-C (d) all of the above

48. Viral infected cells can escape from NK cell mediated killing by expressing

(a) Normal levels of MHC class I

(b) MHC II

(c) High level of ICAMs

(d) High level of Mannose-6-P receptor

49. Target-cell killing by ADCC involves different cytotoxic mechanisms except

(a) Perforins (b) TNF

(c) Lytic enzymes (d) Complement

50. The types of cells involved in ADCC are,

(a) Neutrophil (b) Eosinophil

(c) NK cell (d) Macrophages

(e) All of the above

51. In one way MLR, one population is rendered unresponsive by treatment of

(a) Mitomycin C (b) lethal X-irradiation

(c) both (d) None

52. In MLR the proliferating cells are

(a) T_H cells (b) T_C cells

(c) Macrophages (d) None of the above

53. Cr ^{51}used in CML labels the target cells by binding with

(a) DNA (b) Cytoplasmic Protein

(c) RNA (d) None

54. GVH reaction develops due to,

(a) Attack of grafted lymphocytes on host tissue

(b) Attack of host immune cells on graft tissue

(c) Autoimmunity

(d) Hypersensitivity reaction

55. Spleen enlargement in GVH reaction is due to the proliferation of

(a) $CD4^+$ cells (b) $CD8^+$ cells

(c) Both (d) Macrophages

56. Major organ affected by GVH reaction is
    (a) Liver (b) Spleen
    (c) Lung (d) intestine
57. Apoptosis is characterized by,
    (a) Membrane blebbing
    (b) Flipping of phosphatidylserine in the membrane
    (c) Nuclear fragmentation
    (d) All of the above
58. Which of the following is active process ?
    (a) Apoptosis (b) Necrosis
    (c) both (d) None
59. Macrophage activation mediates _____ types of immune response
    (a) T_H1 (b) T_H2
    (c) both (d) None
60. The cell types involved in T_H2 type of immune response
    (a) Macrophages (b) NK cells
    (c) eosinophils (d) Neutrophil
61. T_H1 and T_H2 subsets can be differentiated by,
    (a) Phenotypic markers (b) Cytokine milieu
    (c) Both (d) None

True or false

62. Effector cells and memory T cells need costimulation.
63. The level of LFA-1 and CD2 is twofold to four fold higher on naive T cells than on effector T cells.
64. Naive Tc cells are capable of killing target cells.

65. IL-2 receptor is expressed on CTL-Ps.
66. Granzymes can directly mediate DNA fragmentation.
67. Apoptotic process by granzymes need protein synthesis.
68. Caspases are present in the cell as active enzymes.
69. CTLs don't kill the target cells as persuade them to commit suicide.
70. T cells and NK cells originate from different progenitor cells.
71. Different NK cells express different sets of membrane molecules.
72. Cell depletion with monoclonal anti-CD16 antibody removes almost all NK-cell activity from peripheral blood.
73. The principal role of CMI is to eliminate cells infected with extra cellular pathogens.
74. Nude mice lack functional NK cell population.
75. Unlike T and B cells, NK cells do not undergo rearrangement of receptor genes.
76. NK cells use different mechanisms to kill target cells to those employed by CTLs
77. NK cells do not bear Fas L.
78. NK cells are constitutively cytotoxic.
79. Recognition of target cells by NK cells is MHC restricted.
80. NK cell activity differ with syngenic and allogenic tumor cells.
81. NK cell response generates immunological memory.
82. Most appropriate model for NK cell target recognition is opposing-signals model.

83. The CD94/NKG2 receptors recognize HLA-E on potential target cells.
84. The inhibitory receptor CD94/NKG2 are not specific to particular HLA allele.
85. KIR receptors are specific for one or a limited number of polymorphic products of particular HLA loci.
86. Unlike B and T cells, NK cells are not limited to expressing a single KIR, but may express several, each specific for different MHC molecule.
87. Signals from activating receptors have veto power over inhibitory receptors.
88. Eosinophils do not contain perforins.
89. Macrophages are unnecessary for MLR to proceed.
90. Cells killed by apoptosis trigger inflammation.
91. In CD8 T cells, different responses are triggered by different levels of stimulation.
92. T cell cytotoxicity can be readily induced by a much lower threshold than cytokine synthesis.
93. Cytotoxic T cell is able to induce apoptosis in any cell it recognizes.
94. CD95 pathway is used primarily to destroy virus-infected cells whereas perforin pathway is used to destroy unwanted T cells.
95. The size of perforation produced on target cell by NK cells is larger than T cells.
96. Granulysin from Tc cells ensures that lysed cells do not release viable bacteria.
97. Subsets of $CD8^+$ T cells have been identified in rodents.
98. $CD8^+$ T cells show a strong preference to Tc1 phenotype.

99. Differentiation into Tc2 requires exposure to high levels of IL-4.
100. All three subsets of $CD8^+$ T cells are cytotoxic.
101. ADCC is faster and efficient than T cell mediated cytotoxicity.
102. ADCC is faster than NK cell mediated killing.
103. M2 cells of macrophages are immunosuppressive and anti-inflammatory.
104. M2 cells produce nitric oxide.
105. The effector phase of T cell response is briefer than antibody response.
106. Cytotoxicity is seen only in the presence of antigen.
107. In general, 5 to 10% of the peak number of cytotoxic T cells produced survive to become memory T cells.
108. Each subset of T_H subset amplifies itself and cross regulates the reciprocal subset.
109. The antibodies stimulated by T_H2 cytokines promote phagocytosis or activate complement efficiently.
110. T_H1 cells express chemokine receptors CCR5 and CXCR3 and T_H2 cells express CCR4 and CCR8.
111. Effector T cells express high levels of L-selectin and CCR7.

Match

112. Match the Soluble factors with source of cell.

1. TH1 cell ---- a. Fas ligand
2. TH2 cell ----- b. TNFβ
3. $CD8^+$ CTL ---- c. CD40L

113. Match the Membrane bound molecules

1. IFNγ, GM-CSF ------ a. CTL
2. IL-4, IL-5, L-6 ------- b. B cell
3. Perforin, granzyme ------- c. TH1

114.

1. *lpr* mice – a. lack of B and T cells
2. *gld* mice – b. mutated CD95
3. Beige mice – c. lack of NK cells
4. Nude mice – d. mutated CD95L

115. 1. STAT 4 – a. TH2

2. STAT 6 – b. TH1
3. T bet – c. TH2
4. GATA 3 – d. TH1

Answers

1. secreted antibodies
2. macrophages, B cells
3. TNF and Fas ligand
4. IL-2
5. Perforin-granzyme and fas
6. mannose 6 phosphate
7. caspase
8. 5-10%
9. Chediak-Higashi
10. CD16
11. Thymic
12. C-type lectin inhibitory receptor, and KIR.
13. HLA-E
14. Mixed lymphocyte reaction (MLR)
15. Cell mediated lympholysis (CML)
16. Graft versus host reaction (GVH)
17. ADCC
18. 1.3
19. IFNγ and TNFα
20. IL-12
21. TNF-α
22. DISC, apoptosome
23. $CD4^+$ IL-2β
24. IL-15 ,IL-2
25. True
26. IFNγ, IL-4
27. Granulysin
28. CLA

29. $\alpha_4\beta_7$
30. d
31. a
32. b
33. d
34. c
35. c
36. c
37. c
38. a
39. a
40. a
41. c
42. b
43. b
44. b
45. c
46. b
47. d
48. a
49. d
50. e
51. c
52. a
53. b
54. a
55. c
56. b
57. d
58. a
59. a
60. c
61. b
62. False
63. False
64. False
65. False
66. False
67. False
68. False
69. True
70. False
71. True
72. True
73. False
74. False
75. True
76. False
77. False
78. True
79. False
80. False
81. False
82. True
83. True
84. True
85. True
86. True
87. False
88. False
89. False
90. False
91. True
92. True
93. True
94. False
95. False
96. True
97. True
98. True

99. True
100. True
101. False
102. True
103. True
104. False
105. True
106. True
107. True
108. True
109. False
110. True
111. False
112. 1.b,2.c,3.a
113. 1.c2.b,3.a
114. 1.b,2.d3.c,4.a
115. 1.b,2.a,3.d,4.c

Chapter 11

Complement system

Fill in the blanks

1. The complement system is the major effector of ___________ branch of the immune system.
2. ___________ identified the presence of complement in serum and ___________ coined the term complement.
3. Half life of C3 convertase C3bBb is increased by the binding of a serum protein ___________.
4. Most mammalian cells have higher levels of ________ that contributes to the rapid inactivation of bound C3b molecules on the host cells.
5. Complement components account for about __________% of the globulin fraction of serum.

Choose the best answer

6. Complement components are

   (a) Soluble proteins (b) Cell-bound proteins

   (c) Both (d) None

7. Basic functions of complement system include,

   (a) Lysis of pathogen (b) Opsonisation

   (c) Inflammation (d) Immune clearance

   (e) All of the above

8. Main source of complement component is

(a) Liver hepatocytes (b) Macrophages

(c) Epithelium of GI tract

(d) Epithelium of urinary tract

9. Which of the following component is larger?

(a) C3 (b) C5

(c) C1 (d) C9

10. At least ________ of the C_1 q globular heads must bind by Fc sites for activation

(a) 2 (b) 4

(c) 6 (d) 8

11. Alternate pathway is initiated by,

(a) Antigen-antibody complex

(b) Cell surface components

(c) Free antibodies

(d) None of above

12. Which of the following has C3 convertase activity ?

(a) C4b2a (b) C3bBb

(c) Both (d) C4b2aBb

13. The first components which initiates the membrane attack complex on the target cell is?

(a) C_5a (b) C5b

(c) C_6 (d) C_9

14. which of the following is most potent anaphylotoxin ?

(a) C_3a (b) C_{4b}

(c) iC_3b (d) None

15. which of the following cell is important in removing immune complexes from circulation ?

(a) RBC (b) Macrophages

(c) Neutrophils (d) Monocytes

16. Which of the following pathway is associated with acquired immunity.

(a) classical (b) alternate

(c) MBL pathway (d) None

17. which of the following component is found in highest concentration in serum ?

(a) C_{19} (b) C_3

(c) C_5 (d) C_9

18. Follicular dendritic cells attach to immune complexes via________receptor.

(a) CR1 (b) CR2

(c) CR3 (d) CR4

True or false

19. Complement components circulate in the serum in functionally active form.

20. Classical pathway of complement begins with formation of antigen-antibody complexes.

21. C_1q is composed of 18 polypeptide chains that associate to form six collagen-like triple helical arms.

22. Circulating free IgM molecules can activate complement.

23. Single molecule of IgM can activate complement pathway whereas 1000 molecules of IgG are required for the same.

24. A single C3 convertase molecule can generate over 200 molecules of C3b.

25. Alternate pathway of complement system is a component of innate immune system.

26. C3bBb3B complex exhibits C5 convertase activity produced in alternate pathway, analogous to the C4b2a3b complex in the classical pathway.
27. Only Gram negative bacteria can activate alternate pathway.
28. The lectin pathway, like the alternative pathway, does not depend on antibody for its activation.
29. MBL is an acute phase protein produced in inflammatory responses.
30. MASP-1 and MASP-2 proteins of MBL pathway have structural similarity to C1r and C1s and mimic their activities.
31. C_5b component is heat stable.
32. The MAC has a functional pore size of 70-100A° .
33. Complement mediated lysis is more effective if the complement is from a species different from that of the cells being lysed.
34. Homologous restriction poses a barrier to the xenotransplantation.
35. All enveloped viruses are susceptible to complement mediated lysis.
36. A single MAC can lyse nucleated cells.
37. Carboxypeptidase N inactivates anaphylotoxins.
38. Deficiencies of C_1, C_2, C_4 and CR1 predispose an individual to SLE.
39. Although RBCs express lower levels of CR1, erythrocytes accounts for about 90% of CR1 is blood.
40. Deficiencies of factor D and properdin are associated with immune complex diseases.
41. Deficiency of C_9 results in clinical symptoms.
42. Patients with C_3 deficiencies have most severe clinical manifestations.

43. Deficiency of C_1 inhibitor gives rise to a condition called hereditary angioedema.
44. C_4 deficient individuals have difficulty in eliminating immune complexes.
45. The complement system is active in healthy, uninfected animals.
46. Neutrophils can store large quantities of C_6 and C_7.
47. IgG is more efficient than IgM in activating the classical pathway.
48. C_{5b67} is chemotactic for neutrophils and eosinophils.
49. Depletion of C_3 is associated with reduced primary antibody responses.
50. C_3 deficient dogs tend to make more IgG and less IgM.
51. Complement is inactivated by heating serum to 56°C for 30 min.
52. Microbes express higher levels of sialic acid than mammalian cells do.
53. Deficiency of DAF results in a disease called Paroxysmal nocturnal hemoglobinuria.
54. Match the regulatory proteins and their mode of action.

    1. C_1 inhibitor - (a) Cleavage of C_3b
    2. Factor H - (b) Blocks binding of MAC
    3. Factor I - (c) dissociates $C_1r_2S_2$
    4. DAF - (d) blocks C_3 convertase
    5. HRF - (e) Decay of C_3 convertase

55. Define

Substrate modulation

This is one way of regulation of complement system. The target for a protease is not susceptible to cleavage unless it is first bound to another protein. e.g. C_1 can act upon C_2, only after it binds to $C_{4r}b$.

Answers

1. humoral
2. Jules Bordet, Paul Ehrich
3. properdin
4. sialic acid
5. 15%
6. c
7. e
8. a
9. c
10. a
11. b
12. c
13. b
14. a
15. a
16. a
17. b
18. a
19. False
20. True
21. True
22. False
23. True
24. True
25. True
26. True
27. False
28. True
29. True
30. True
31. False
32. True
33. True
34. True
35. True
36. False
37. True
38. True
39. True
40. False
41. False
42. True
43. True
44. True
45. False
46. True
47. False
48. True
49. True
50. False
51. True
52. False
53. True
54. 1.c, 2.d, 3.a, 4.e, 5.b

Chapter 12

Cytokines

Fill in the blanks

1. __________ cytokine is required for the final maturation of B cells into plasma cells.
2. _________ is an immunosuppressive and anti-inflammatory cytokine.
3. _________ cytokine aids in the transition of innate immunity to acquired immunity.
4. Class I cytokine receptor family have conserved four cysteine residues and a conserved sequence of __________.
5. Two transcriptional factors, _______ and _______ are key elements indetermining subset commitment and cross-regulation.
6. Although less than 0.01% of T cells respond to a given conventional antigen, between _____to_______% of T cells can respond to a given super antigen.
7. The two major families of chemokines are _____ family in which the cysteine residues are adjacent, and the ______ family, in which these residues are separated by one amino acid.

Choose the best answer

8. IL-26 is produced by

(a) Activated T cells (b) Naive T cells

(c) Memory T cells (d) B cells

9. Specificity of cytokines is maintained by following ways except

   (a) regulation of expression of cytokine receptors on cells

   (b) Half life of cytokines is very short

   (c) produced only by antigen activated immune cells

   (d) acts in antigen specific manner

10. The receptors for hematopoietins belong to

    (a) Class I cytokine receptor family

    (b) Class II cytokine receptor family

    (c) TNF receptor family

    (d) Ig super family

11. T cell activation antigen represents which subunit of IL-2 receptor ?

    (a) α (b) β

    (c) γ (d) $\beta\gamma$

12. Which of following plays a central role in immune regulation ?

    (a) IFN α (b) IFN β

    (c) IFN γ (d) IFN λ.

True or false

13. Cells secrete only one cytokine at a time.

14. Chemokines primarily act as chemotactic factors and leukocyte activators.

15. IL-1RA has anti-inflammatory effects.

16. Only Th1 cells produce IL-2.
17. TNF-α receptors are found on almost all nucleated cells.
18. T cells have both high affinity and low affinity IL-2 receptors.
19. B cells have about 1000 high affinity receptors and 10,000 low affinity receptors.
20. INF-γ stimulates B cell production of IgG2a.
21. IL-4 enhances the development of cytotoxic T cells from resting T cells and can make helper T cells grow in the absence of IL-2.
22. Both IL-4 and IFN-γ enhance MHC II expression in macrophages.
23. IL-9 is a stem cell growth factor produced only by Th2 cells.
24. IL-13 induces differentiation of Th cells.
25. Activated memory T cells produce IL-17.
26. The receptor for IL-16 is CD4.
27. IL-12 stimulates naive Th1 cells, whereas IL-23 stimulates Th1 memory cells.
28. IL-28, 29, 30 are known as λ interferons.
29. IFN-α is a potent stimulator of adaptive immunity only.
30. IL-15 shares many biological activities with IL-2.
31. TGF-β induces T and B cell proliferation.
32. Th3 cells are activated $CD4^+$ T cells secreting large amounts of TGF-β.
33. Most of the virokines tend to be antiviral immuno-suppressive molecules.
34. Cytokines are produced constitutively.

35. Cytokines generally have a molecular mass of less than 30 kDa.

36. The two principal producers of cytokines are T_H cell and macrophages.

37. Cytokines act in an antigen specific manner.

38. *In vivo*, cytokines rarely act alone.

39. The class II cytokine receptors lack the WSXWS motif.

40. NK cells express β and γ subunits of IL-2 R constitutively.

41. Class I and II cytokine receptors lack signaling motifs.

42. IL-RA binds to IL-1 receptor but has no activity.

43. The presence of soluble IL-2R has been used as a clinical marker of recent T cell activation.

44. The array of cytokines secreted by $CD8^+$ CTLs is generally wider than that of CD4+ T_H cells.

45. Both TH1 and TH2 subsets secrete IL-3 and GM-CSF.

46. TH2 subset activates non complement activating IgG isotypes.

47. The generation of TH2 cells depends critically on IL-4.

48. IFN -γ preferentially inhibits proliferation of TH2 subset.

49. All cytokine binding receptors contain two or three subunits.

50. Expression of the β subunit of IL-2 receptor is indicative of T cell activation.

51. All members of each subfamily of the class I cytokine receptors share a common signal transducing subunit.

52. All chemokines are 8 to 12 kd polypeptides that contain two internal disulfide loops.

53. IL-12 is a key inducer of cell-mediated immunity.

54. IL-10 induces the expression of co stimulators and MHC II on macrophages and dendritic cells.

55. IL-18 is structurally homologous to IL-1.

56. IL-2 is a growth factor and responsible for T cell clonal expansion.

57. IL-2 potentiates apoptotic death of antigen activated T cells.

58. TGF β stimulates production of IgE antibodies by inducing B cells to switch to this isotype.

59. IL-3 is known as multilineage colony-stimulating factor.

Match

60.

(1) IL-4 and IL-5 – (a) Antagonism

(2) IL-4 and IFN-γ – (b) redundancy

(3) IL-4 – (c) Synergy

(4) IL-4,IL-2,IL-5 – (d) Pleiotrophy

61.

(1) Group I cytokines – (a) cell death

(2) Group II cytokines – (b) inflammation

(3) Group III cytokines – (c) hematopoiesis

62.

(1) IFN-ω – (a) Pig trophoblast

(2) IFN-τ – (b) human, horse, dog trophoblast

(3) IFN-δ – (c) ruminant trophoblast

63. Differnetiate cytokines and harmones

Cytokines	**Harmones**
a. Act over a short distance	Act long range
b. Often produced by and bind to a variety of cells	Produced by specialized glands and tend to have a unique action on one or few types of target cell

Answers

1. IL-6
2. IL-10
3. IL-21
4. WSXWS
5. T-Bet and GATA-3
6. 5% to 25%
7. CC ,CXC
8. c
9. d
10. a
11. a
12. c
13. False
14. True
15. True
16. True
17. True
18. False
19. True
20. True
21. True
22. True
23. True
24. False
25. True
26. True
27. True
28. True
29. False
30. True
31. False
32. True
33. True
34. True
35. True
36. True
37. False
38. True
39. True
40. True
41. True
42. True
43. False
44. False
45. True
46. True
47. True
48. True

49. False
50. False
51. True
52. True
53. True
54. False
55. True
56. True
57. True
58. False
59. True
60. 1.c, 2.a, 3.d,4.b
61. 1.c, 2.a, 3.b
62. 1.b, 2.c, 3.a

Chapter 13

Microbial immunity

Fill in the blanks

1. __________ cells frequently form the first line of defense against viral infections.
2. The activity of NK cells is greatly enhanced by __________ cytokine.
3. The current vaccine for tuberculosis consists of an attenuated strain of *M. bovis* called ___________.
4. Variation in influenza surface proteins is generated by __________ and ______________.
5. The diptheria vaccine is a formaldehyde treated preparation of the exotoxin, called a______________.
6. The primary host defense against viral and bacterial attachment to epithelial surfaces is ___________.

Choose the best answer

7. Bacterial HSPs are highly antigenic because

   (a) They are produced in abundance in infected host.

   (b) Readily processed by APCs

   (c) Large no. of immune cells respond to HSP

   (d) All of the above

8. Which of following are induced by interferons following viral infection

   (a) 2'5' oligoadenylate synthetase

(b) Protein kinase

(c) Mx proteins

(d) Nitric oxide synthase

(e) All of the above

True or false

9. Viruses are well known for the stimulation of innate responses.
10. The humoral immune response is the main protective response against intracellular bacteria.
11. Innate immunity is not very effective against intracellular bacterial pathogens.
12. *Neisseria meningitidis* secrete proteases that cleave secretory IgA at hinge region.
13. Variation in pilin, which is expressed by many gram negative bacteria, is generated by the process of gene conversion.
14. Antimicrobial immunity consists of an early innate response followed by a more sustained adaptive response.
15. Bacterial cell walls, lacking sialic acid activates alternate complement pathway.
16. *L. monocytogenes* can travel from cell to cell without exposure to the extra cellular fluid.
17. Lepromatous leprosy is characterized by very high antibody levels and poor cell-mediated responses.
18. Agglutination by antiflagellar antibodies produce fluffy cotton like floccules whereas that of somatic antigens produce fine granular clumps.
19. Interferons are glycoproteins.

20. IFN-τ has been isolated from ruminant trophoblast, and IFN δ has been isolated from pig trophoblast.
21. IFN *k* is another name for IL-28.
22. The type I interferons are not stable at pH 2, whereas IFN γ is stable.
23. Kidney cells are poor interferon producers and neutrophils produce no interferon.
24. In antibacterial immunity, IgG is quantitatively the most significant immunoglobulin, whereas IgM is qualitatively superior.
25. Interferons are virus specific.
26. Herpes viruses and poxviruses express IL-10 cytokine homolog that suppress Th1 responses.
27. Haemagglutination - inhibition are not strain -specific.
28. Eimeria infection generally leads to strong species specific immunity that can prevent reinfection.
29. Helminths replicate within a host like protozoa.
30. Helminths usually cause morbidity but not mortality.
31. The eotaxins have selective chemotactic activity for eosinophils.

Match

32.

1. Influenza virus --a. Type 2 complement receptor
2. Rhinovirus -- b. Sialic acid residues
3. Epstein-Barr virus -- c. ICAM

33. Match the immune evasion strategies with specific virus.

1. EBV --- a. Downregulation of MHC I
2. Paramyxo Vs --- b. Immunosuppression

3. Rhino Vs ---- c. BCRF 1

4. Adeno Vs ---- d. Antigenic variation

Define

34. Antigenic drift

Involved a series of spontaneous point mutations that occur gradually, resulting in minor changes of viral surface proteins like HA and neuraminidase.

35. Antigenic shift

Results in sudden emergence of new subtype of virus by reassortment of genome segments.

36. Preimmunity and self-cure phenomenon

Answers

1. NK
2. IL-12
3. BCG
4. antigenic drift and antigenic shift
5. toxoid
6. Secretory IgA
7. d
8. e
9. True
10. False
11. True
12. True
13. True
14. True
15. False
16. True
17. True
18. True
19. True
20. True
21. True
22. False
23. True
24. True
25. False
26. True
27. False
28. True
29. False
30. True
31. True
32. 1.b, 2.c, 3.a
33. 1.c, 2.b, 3.d, 4.a

Chapter 14

Vaccines

Fill in the blanks

1. An international unit (U) of tetanus immunoglobulin is the specific neutralizing activity contained in ______ mg of the international standard.
2. To reduce antigenicity, the immunoglobulins are usually treated with ______ enzyme that leaves intact $F(ab)'_2$ fragment for neutralization.
3. ______ is a rough mutant of *B. abortus* used in vaccination recently.
4. Examples of alkylating agents include ________ , ________ and __________.
5. First commercially available category I recombinant veterinary vaccine was made against _______.
6. Good, effective vaccines should have a PF of at least _______%
7. The first recombinant antigen vaccine approved for human use is________.
8. _________ are lipid carriers prepared by mixing protein with detergent and a glycoside called quill A.

Choose the best answer

9. The limitations of DNA vaccine are

   (a) Activate oncogenes

(b) Anti-nuclear antibodies

(c) Antibiotic resistance

(d) All of the above

True or false

10. Passive immunization is most effective in protection against toxigenic bacteria.
11. Formaldehyde cross-links proteins and nucleic acids and confers structural rigidity.
12. DNA vaccines are not able to induce immunity in the presence of very high titers of maternal antibody.
13. DNA vaccine delivered via Gene gun preferentially stimulates a Th2 response.
14. Viral DNA in eye drops can induce an IgA response in the tears and bile of recipients.
15. Depot adjuvants influence only the primary immune response and have little effect on secondary immune response.
16. Aluminium based adjuvants have good stimulatory effect on cell-mediated immune responses.
17. LPS has immunostimulatory activity, but have no effect on cell-mediated responses.
18. Saponin based adjuvants may selectively stimulate Th1 activity.
19. FCA promotes IgG production over IgM.
20. FCA inhibits tolerance induction, favors DTH, accelerates graft rejection and promotes resistance to tumors.
21. FCA is acceptable in food animals.
22. Vaccine Doses are formulated to account for body weight or age.

23. Heavily parasitized or malnourished animals should not be vaccinated.
24. Trypsinization of the ana culture makes it more immunogenic.
25. Passive immunization activates the immune system and generates memory response.
26. Vaccination is 100% effective.
27. Killed vaccines are less effective in inducing CMI and secretory IgA response than live attenuated vaccines.
28. Polysaccharide vaccines are unable to activate T_H cells.
29. Unlike vaccinia, the canarypox virus does not appear to be virulent even in individuals with severe immune suppression.
30. ISCOMS induce cell-mediated immune response.
31. Multivalent subunit vaccines generally induce a greater response than synthetic peptide vaccines.
32. DNA vaccines don't generate significant immunologic memory.
33. A DNA vaccine only induces a response to a single epitope.

Match

34.

1. Strain 19 – (a) *B. ovis*
2. Strain 45/20 – (b) Rough mutant
3. Rev. 1 – (c) live attenauted
4. RB-51 – (d) killed

35.

1. First marker vaccine -- (a) Rabies
2. First recombinant antigen for vaccine –(b) Pseudo rabies

3. First use of viral vector for vaccine – (c) FMD

Define

36. Anaculture

Some vaccines combine both toxoid and killed bacteria in a single dose by the simple expedient of formolizing a whole cutlure. These products are known as anacultures.

37. SMAA : Solid matrix antigen - antibody complexes are made by attaching monoclonal antibodies to particulate solid matrices and then saturating the antibody with the desired antigen. The resulting complexes are then used as vaccines. By attaching different monoclonal antibodies to the solid matrix, it is possible to bind a mixture of peptides or proteins, composing immunodominant epitopes for both T cells and B cells to the solid matrix. These multivalent complexes have been shown to induce vigorous humoral and CMI responses.

38. Reverse vaccinology

Now the complete genomes of pathogens are avaialble hence it is possible to identify potential vaccine antigen by computer analysis. This can rapidly identify novel potential vaccine candidates.

39. Herd immunity

Herd immunity is the resistance of an entire group of animals to a disease as a result of the presence, in that group, of a proportion of immune animals.

40. Ring vaccination : Seeks to contain an outbreak by establishing a barrier of immune animals around an infected area.

41. Predictive vaccination : Seeks to vaccinate the animals on farms likely to contribute most to the future spread of disease.

42. Preventable fraction (PF):

$$PF = \frac{\%\text{ of controls dying} - \%\text{ of vaccinates dying}}{\%\text{ of controls dying}}$$

43. DIVA : Differentiate infected from vaccinated animals.

44. Mixed modality vaccine

45. Prime boost vaccine

Answers

1. 0.03384
2. Pepsin
3. RB-51
4. ethylene oxide, β-propionolactone and acetyl ethyleneimine.
5. feline leukemia virus
6. 80%
7. hepatitis B vaccine
8. ISCOMS
9. d
10. True
11. True
12. False
13. True
14. True
15. True
16. False
17. True
18. True
19. True
20. True
21. False
22. False
23. True
24. True
25. False
26. False
27. True
28. True
29. True
30. True
31. True
32. False
33. False
34. 1.c,2.d,3.a,4.b
35. 1.b,2.c,3.a

Chapter 15

Mucosal Immuntiy

Fill in the blanks

1. IgA class switching is stimulated by cytokine _______ and ________
2. FcRn is unique among Fc receptors in that it resembles __________ molecule.
3. Enteric defensins produced by paneth cells known as ________ prevent bacteria from entering the crypts.
4. Lactoferrin in milk competes with bacteria for _______ and makes it unavailable for their growth.
5. ________ are the largest of the mucosal lymphoid tissues.
6. At mucosal surfaces IgM and IgA act by _________ whereas, the IgE and IgG, destroy antigen within the surface tissues by _________.

Choose the best answer

7. At mucosal sites, the principal mechanism of protective immunity is provided by

   (a) lymphocytes (b) antibodies

   (c) phagocytes (d) complement

8 The first lymphoid organ to develop in a newborn is

   (a) thymus (b) spleen

   (c) lymph nodes (d) mucosal lymphoid tissues

9. In hemochorial type of placenta which isotype is transferred to the fetus ?

    (a) IgA (b) IgM

    (c) IgG (d) IgE

10. Transfer of immunoglobulin via placenta is completely absent in which species?

    (a) horse (b) dog

    (c) primate (d) cat

11. Predominating lymphocytes in colostrum is

    (a) T (b) B

    (c) NK cells (d) None

True or false

12. IL-5 producing T-helper cells are more numerous in mucosal than in other lymphoid tissues.
13. Transport of maternal for IgG across the placenta and across the neonatal intestinal epithelium is mediated by neonatal Fc receptor FcRn.
14. Interaction of IgG with FcRn involves peptide binding cleft of MHC I molecule.
15. Knockout mice lacking β2-microglobulin have 10 fold lower levels of serum IgG than normal mice.
16. Gnotobiotic animals have well developed secondary lymphoid organs.
17. Bovine cryptidins are secreted in inactive precursor form.
18. Lactoferrin is apparently able to substitute for antibodies and activate C_{1q}.
19. Spleen contains more lymphocytes than intestine.

20. Jejunal Peyer's patches are primary lymphoid organs whereas ileocecal peyer's patches are secondary lymphoid organs.
21. The proportion of M cells in the follicle associated with epithelium varies from 10% in humans and mice to 50% in rabbits and to 100% in terminal ileum of pigs and calves.
22. MadCAM-1 is expressed only on the high endothelial venules of Peyer's patches and on venules in intestinal lamina propria and the mammary gland.
23. The CD8 molecules on the IELs consists of α/α homodimers rather than α/β heterodimer.
24. IEL T cells originate within the bone marrow and mature within cryptopatches.
25. IELs lack proliferative response due to the absence of CD5 and CD28.
26. Th1 cells are the predominant helper cells found in surface tissues.
27. The production, transport and secretion of secretory component occurs only in the presence of IgA.
28. IgA is not bactericidal and activates complement only by the alternate and lectin pathways.
29. In rats, rabbits and chickens bile is the major source of IgA.
30. In major domestic mammals less than 5% of IgA enters the bile.
31. S IgA is much more susceptible to proteases than s IgM.
32. Cells producing IgE are mainly found in lymph nodes or spleen.
33. More than 80% of the body's activated B cells are found in the intestine.

34. Oral tolerance may involve either cellular suppression or clonal anergy and is greatly directed against Th1 cells.

35. IgA is locally synthesized in the mammary tissue, whereas IgG is actively transported from serum to milk.

36. The predominant immunoglobulin in cervico-vaginal mucus is IgG, whereas within the uterus it is IgA.

37. The lungs of the majority of domestic species differ from rodent, human or dog lungs in that they contain large number of intravascular macrophages.

38. Multiple doses of vaccine may not increase the intensity or duration of local immune response.

39. When a chick hatches it possess IgY in its serum and IgM and IgA in its intestine.

40. IgM and IgA of albumin in fertilized egg are actively transported from hen's serum.

41. All antigens are equally capable of stimulating fetal lymphoid tissue.

42. B cells can be found in the thymus of new born pigs.

43. Development of humoral immune responses in dog is earlier than other domestic animals.

44. Macrophages from neonatally thymectomized mice do not acquire virucidal activity.

45. In newborn piglet 75% of particles are cleared from the liver and spleen whereas in adult it is carried out by alveolar macrophages.

46. Any immunoglobulin in the serum of a newborn unsuckled animal suggests infection in utero.

47. In pigs and horses, IgA predominates in colostrum and IgG in milk.

48. All the IgG, most of the IgM and about half of the IgA in bovine colostrum are derived from serum.
49. Ruminants selectively absorbs the immunoglobulin classes.
50. In horse and pigs IgA is not absorbed and remains in intestine of neonates.
51. Colostrum is full of lymphocytes.
52. Measles vaccine given to puppies at 6 weeks of age may induce a protective response in spite of high levels of anti-distemper HA antibody.

Answers

1. TGF-β and IL-5
2. MHC I
3. Cryptdins
4. Iron
5. Peyer's patches
6. Immune exclusion , immune elimination
7. b
8. a
9. c
10. a
11. a
12. True
13. True
14. False
15. True
16. False
17. False
18. True
19. False
20. False
21. True
22. True
23. True
24. True
25. True
26. False
27. False
28. True
29. True
30. True
31. False
32. False
33. True
34. True
35. True
36. False
37. True
38. True
39. True
40. False
41. False
42. True
43. False

44. True
45. True
46. True
47. False
48. True
49. False
50. True
51. True
52. True

Chapter 16

Tolerance/ Immuno Regulation

Fill in the blanks

1. ________ is the specific immunological unresponsiveness of an individual to an antigen.
2. T cells can be made tolerant rapidly and easily when compared to B cells.
3. ________ is a major mechanism of self tolerance.
4. Very high doses of an antigen can also induce a form of clonal anergy called ________.
5. An excellent example of an inhibitory receptor is ________.
6. The immune system signals the central nervous system through ________.
7. Antigens that induce tolerance are called ________.
8. ________producing B cells are much more readily suppressed than those producing IgG or IgM.

Choose the best answer

9. Fading of tolerance can be hastened by

   (a) Low-dose irradiation (b) Removal of antigen

   (c) Metabolism of antigen (d) All of the above

10. Which of the following is not a B cell inhibitory receptor ?

    (a) CD5 (b) CD22

(c) CD72 (d) CD66a

(e) CD21

11. Regulatory T cells are

(a) $CD4^+$ cells (b) $CD8^+$ cells

(c) $CD4^+$, $CD25^+$ cells (d) $CD8^+$ $CD25^+$ cells

12. Which of the following stage is more sensitive for tolerance induction ?

(a) CD^{4+} (b) CD^{8+}

(c) Double positive stage (d) Double negative stage

True or false

13. Negative selection is a perfect process.
14. Clonal abortion occurs only if B cells encounter an antigen early in their development within the bone marrow.
15. Orally administered proteins may not induce tolerance.
16. High doses of antigen induce clonal deletion and anergy whereas lower doses induce the development of regulatory cells.
17. B cells, like T cells do not undergo receptor editing.
18. Acquired immune responses are not antigen driven.
19. Antigens that do not reach organized lymphoid tissues, fail to induce either an immune response or tolerance.
20. DC1 cells are optimized to present antigens to Th1 cells whereas DC2 cells present antigens to Th2 cells.
21. IgG antibodies suppress the production of both IgM and IgG whereas IgM antibodies tend to suppress only further synthesis of IgM.

22. Specific antibodies tend to suppress a specific immune response better than nonspecific immuno globulins.
23. Regulatory T cells secrete IL-10 and TGF-β cytokine to suppress other T cell responses.
24. IL-10 inhibits not only Th1 but also many Th2 responses.
25. IDO from dendritic cells is a potent inhibitor of T cell proliferation and survival.
26. α-endorphin suppresses antibody formation and β-endorphin reverses this suppressive effect.
27. Photoperiod do not influence immune responses.
28. Tolerance is immunologically non-specific.
29. TGF-β is an inhibitor of T cell and B cell proliferation.
30. IL-10 antagonizes the actions of the principal macrophage activating cytokine IFN-γ.
31. High doses of antigens administered systemically without adjuvants tend to induce tolerance.

Define

32. Central tolerance

Central tolerance occurs during their maturation in the generative lymphoid organs, all lymphocytes pass through a stage in which encounter with antigen leads to tolerance rather than activation.

33. Peripheral tolerance

Peripheral tolerance is induced when mature lymphocytes recognize antigens without adequate levels of co stimulators that are required for activation or as a result of persistent and repeated stimulation by self antigens in peripheral tissues.

34. Receptor editing

    B cells in the bone marrow that encounter self antigens instead of destroyed by apoptosis, respond to these antigens by reactivating their RAG1 and RAG2 genes and expressing a new Ig light chain, thus acquiring a new specificity. This process is called receptor editing.

35. Clonal energy

    The prolonged, antigen-specific suppression of T cell function, due to lack of co stimulatory signals delivered to a T or B cell is known as clonal anergy.

Answers

1. Tolerance
2. True
3. Clonal deletion
4. immune paralysis
5. CD32-B1
6. cytokines
7. Tolerogens
8. IgE
9. d
10. e
11. b
12. c
13. False
14. True
15. False
16. True
17. False
18. False
19. True
20. True
21. True
22. True
23. True
24. True
25. True
26. True
27. False
28. False
29. True
30. True
31. True

Chapter 17

Clinical immunology

Fill in the blanks

1. Serum can be depleted of complement activity by heating to ______ for ______minutes.
2. __________ test is a gel diffusion method used to detect antibodies against equine infectious anemia virus in horse serum.
3. _________ test is a form of neutralization test carried out entirely *in vivo*.
4. The affinity constant can be determined by _____________.
5. Give Scatchard equation ____________.
6. _________ assay allows quantitative determination of the number of cell in a population that are producing antibodies specific for a given antigen.

Choose the best answer

7. Which of the following test is most sensitive ?

   (a) ELISA (b) RIA

   (c) FAT (d) IPT

8. Enzymes are preferable over radioisotopes for labeling because,

   (a) Isotopes have short half life.

   (b) Potentially hazardous

(c) Require expensive detection devices.

(d) All of the above

9. The ratio of antibody to antigen is optimal at

   (a) Prozone (b) Zone of equivalence

   (c) Post zone (d) None

10. In prozone,

    (a) Antigen is excess (b) Antibody is excess

    (c) Both are excess (d) Both are optimum

11. Which of the following test is used in diagnosis of congenital deficiency of some serum proteins ?

    (a) Immunoelectrophoresis (b) RIA

    (c) ELISA (d) IPT

12. Incomplete antibodies lack agglutinating activity because

    (a) epitopes with which they react lie deep

    (b) restricted movement of hinge region

    (c) both (d) None

13. Isotype efficient in precipitation is

    (a) IgG (b) IgM

    (c) IgA (d) IgE

True or false

14. Primary binding tests directly measure the binding of antigen to antibody are more sensitive than secondary binding tests.

15. Complement in fresh, unheated guinea pig serum is the most efficient in hemolytic tests.

16. ELISAs can be used to test fluids other than blood also.

17. Horse antibodies produce a distinct flocculation over a very narrow range of antigen concentration.
18. Soluble antigen agglutinates specific antibody.
19. Radial immunodiffusion is an quantitative test.
20. Agglutination is more sensitive than precipitation.
21. Neutralization tests are highly specific and extremely sensitive.
22. Highly sensitive tests tend to be relatively nonspecific and highly specific tests are generally insensitive.
23. Valency is the total number of binding sites per antibody molecules.
24. Antibodies that aggregate soluble antigens are called precipitins.
25. Direct ELISA is more sensitive than indirect ELISA.
26. For precipitation to occur, both antigen and antibody must be multivalent.
27. ELISA tests using chromoges are more sensitive than chemiluminescence.
28. Western blotting and immunoprecipitation assays are quantitative assays.
29. Affinity of an antibody is a better measure than its avidity.
30 Usually, if a few hundred copies of a gene are injected into pronuclei about 25% of the mice that are born are transgenic.
31. **Define** - Titre

    The reciprocal of the highest dilution giving a positive reaction, called the titre, provides an estimate of the amount of antibody in the serum.
32. **Define** - Affinity

The combined strength of the noncovalent interactions between a single antigen binding site on an antibody and a single epitope is the affinity of the antibody for that epitope.

33. **Define** - Avidity

The overall strength of interaction between a single antibody molecule to an antigen is known as avidity.

Answers

1. 56^oC for 30 minutes.
2. Coggins
3. Protection
4. equilibrium dialysis
5. $r/c = K_a n - K_a r$
6. ELISPOT
7. b
8. d
9. b
10. b
11. a
12. c
13. a
14. True
15. True
16. True
17. True
18. False
19. True
20. True
21. True
22. True
23. True
24. True
25. False
26. True
27. False
28. False
29. False
30. True

Chapter 18

Immunomodulation

Fill in the blanks

1. Corticosteroids suppress the ability of T cells to produce all cytokines except ________.

2. Examples of newly developed immunosuppressive drugs are, __________ and ___________.

3. Acemannan, derived from *Aloe vera* plant is enhancer of cytokine synthesis, with _________ and ________ activities.

Choose the best answer

4. Corticosteroids influence immunity via.

   (a) altering leukocyte circulation

   (b) altering inflammatory mediators

   (c) modify protein, carbohydrate, fat metabolism

   (d) all of the above

5. Corticosteroids has no effect upon

   (a) lymphocytes (b) macrophages

   (c) neutrophils (d) complement

True or false

6. Laboratory rodents and humans are much more sensitive to the corticosteroid immunosuppression than the major domestic animals.

7. In horses and cattle the no. of circulating eosinophils, basophils and lymphocytes declines abruptly upon corticosteroid administration.
8. T-cells tend to be corticosteroid resistant.
9. Corticosteroids potentiates the action of cyclophosphamide.
10. Azathioprine is useful in control of allograft rejection but in ineffective against xenograft rejection.
11. The combination of corticosteroids and cyclosporine is potent and enhances survival of allograft.
12. Killed *Propionibacterium acne* promote antibody formation.
13. CpG nucleotides when administered alone, greatly enhance innate immunity.
14. Levamisole function in similar manner to thymopoietin.
15. Levamisole has immunomodulating effect on healthy animals.
16. Vitamin E promotes B cell proliferation.
17. Glucocorticoids increase the ability of animals to produce interferon.

Match

18.

1. X-rays	----	(a) Purine analog
2. Corticosteroids	----	(b) Folic acid antagonist
3. Cyclophosphamide	----	(c) Alkylation of DNA
4. Azathioprine	----	(d) ionization
5. Methotrexate	----	(e) NFkB inhibitor

Answers

1. IL-2
2. Mycophenolate mofetil and 15 deoxyspergualin
3. antitumor and antiviral
4. d
5. d
6. True
7. True
8. False
9. False
10. True
11. True
12. True
13. True
14. True
15. False
16. True
17. False
18. 1.d,2.e,3.c,4.a,5.b

Chapter 19

Immunodeficiency disease

Fill in the blanks

1. __________ syndrome involves defect in cytoskeletal glycoprotein present in lymphoid cells called sialophorin.
2. ________ mice are a strain of hairless mice that fail to develop a functional thymus.
3. Starvation-induced immunosuppression is likely mediated through the harmone ________.

Choose the best answer

4. The defect in X linked hyper IgM syndrome is in

   (a) CD40 (b) CD40L

   (c) CD28 (d) CD80

True or false

5. Primary immunodeficiency results from genetic or developmental defect in the immune system.
6. Primary immunodeficiency affects only adaptive immune functions.
7. Reticular dysgenesis affects maturation of all leukocytes.

8. T cell deficiency can affect both humoral and the cell-mediated responses.
9. ADA deficiency results in accumulation of adenosine, which interferes with purine metabolism and DNA synthesis.
10. CD40-CD40L interaction is essential in the generation of germinal centre.
11. In common variable immunodeficiency patients B cells fail to mature into plasma cells.
12. Congenital neutropenias are much more common than acquired ones.
13. Phagocytes from patients with Chediak-Higashi syndrome contain giant granules but do not have the ability to kill bacteria.
14. Leukocyte-adhesion deficiency, causes susceptibility to infection of gram-negative bacteria only.
15. Nude mice can permanently tolerate both allografts and xenografts.
16. Nude mice completely lack T cells.
17. The decrease in $CD4^+$ T cells is the hallmark of AIDS.
18. Most vaccines prevent disease, not infection.
19. The majority of successful vaccines use live-attenuated or heat-killed organisms.
20. X linked agammaglobulinemia (XLA) is a combined B cell and T cell immunodeficiency disease.
21. The hallmark of a phagocytic deficiency is increased susceptibility to viral infections.
22. In chronic granulomatous disease, the underlying defect is in cytochrome or an associated protein.

23. Children born with SCID often manifest increased infections by encapsulated bacteria in the first months of life.
24. Bare lymphocyte syndrome affects cell mediated immunity only.
25. HIV-1 and HIV-2 are more closely related to each other than to SIV.
26. HIV-1 causes immune suppression in both humans and chimpanzees.
27. T cell activation increases transcription of the HIV proviral genome.
28. Patients with advanced stages of AIDS always have detectable antibody to HIV.
29. Pelger-Huet anomaly is an inherited disorder characterized by a failure of granulocyte nuclei to segment into lobes.
30. BLAD calves show delayed or poor type IV responses to intradermal skin testing.
31. Birds of the hypothyroid OS strain have a selective IgA deficiency.
32. Nude mice possess normal numbers of NK cells.
33. Moth-eaten mice have a defective T cell system but produce excessive quantities of immunoglobulins and develop autoimmune disease.
34. FOCMA antigen is expressed on normal cells and also on cells infected with FeLV or FeSV.
35. In general severe nutritional deficiencies reduce T cell function but spare B cell function.
36. Malnutrition increase resistance to viruses.
37. Regular moderate exercise boosts immune function.
38. The bone marrow is relatively unaffected by old age.

Answers

1. Wiskott-Aldrich
2. Nude
3. leptin
4. b
5. True
6. False
7. True
8. True
9. True
10. True
11. True
12. False
13. True
14. False
15. True
16. False
17. False
18. True
19. True
20. False
21. False
22. True
23. False
24. False
25. False
26. False
27. True
28. False
29. True
30. True
31. True
32. True
33. True
34. False
35. True
36. True
37. True
38. True

Chapter 20

Hypersensitivity

Fill in the blanks

1. The term `anaphylaxis' is coined by ________ and ________.
2. Classification of hypersensitivity reactions into four types was proposed by ________ and ________.
3. Sensitized mast cells and basophils are coated by _____ antibody isotype.
4. A hereditary predisposition to the development of immediate hypersensitivity reactions against common environmental antigens is known as ________.
5. The local wheal and flare response that occurs when an allergen is injected into a sensitized individual is called ______ reaction.
6. Hypo sensitization cause shift of IgE towards _______ isotype, and is referred as blocking antibody.
7. Hemolytic diseases of newborn can be entirely prevented by administering Rh antibodies to the mother within 24-48 h after first delivery. These antibodies are known as ________.
8. The hallmark of type IV reaction is recruitment of ________ cells.
9. __________ is the prototype for systemic immune complex-mediated disorders.

Choose the best answer

10. Which of the following is a primary mediator ?

    (a) histamine (b) Leukotriene

    (c) Prostaglandins (d) Cytokines

11. The animal model of choice for studying systemic anaphylaxis is

    (a) Mice (b) Rabbit

    (c) Rat (d) Guinea pig

12. Which cell play a principal role in late -phase reaction?

    (a) Neutrophil (b) Eosinophil

    (c) Basophil (d) Macrophage

13. Type I hypersensitivity can be identified and assessed by

    (a) Skin testing (b) RAST

    (c) RIST (d) PCA

    (e) All of the above

14. Type I hypersensitivity can be controlled by

    (a) avoiding contact with allergen (b) hyposensitisation

    (c) humanised mab-IgE (d) all of the above

15. Hemolytic disease due to Rh incompatibility during pregnancy can be treated by

    (a) blood exchange transfusion (b) low level UV light

    (c) plasmapheresis (d) all of the above

16. In CBH, the predominant cell type is

    (a) Neutrophil (b) Basophil

    (c) Eosinophil (d) Macrophages

True or false

17. Hypersensitivity is an appropriate immune response to an antigen.
18. Hypersensitivity occurs only in the course of humoral immune response.
19. Atopy is multigenic.
20. Low affinity IgE receptor belongs to immunoglobulin super family.
21. Monovalent allergens can crosslink the fixed IgE to trigger degranulation.
22. Histamine exerts negative feedback on the release of mediators on mast cells and basophils.
23. Histamine is more potent than leukotrienes.
24. IL4 increase IgE production by B cells.
25. IL-5 is especially important in the recruitment and activation of eosinophils.
26. Epinephrine is the drug of choice for systemic anaphylactic reactions.
27. Penicillin is notable in that it can induce all four types of hypersensitivity.
28. Much of the tissue damage in type III reactions stems from release of lytic enzymes by neutrophils.
29. DTH response is always detrimental.
30. Antihistamines are effective for the treatment of type III hypersensitivity.
31. Most pollen allergens contain a single allergenic component.
32. Babies can acquire IgE mediated allergies by passive transfer of maternal antibody.

33. Transfusion reactions are a manifestation of type II hypersensitivity.
34. Half life of cell bound IgE is longer than free antibody in serum.
35. FcЄRII is also a ligand for the complement receptor CR2.
36. Basophils are terminally differentiated granulocytes, are not mast cell precursor.
37. Eosinophil peroxidase uses bromide in preference to chloride.
38. In cattle, the major shock organ is the lung.
39. Epinephrine potentiates histamine release in bovine.
40. Dogs differ from the other domestic animals in that the major shock organ is not the lung but the liver.
41. IL-10 inhibits IgE production, mast cell activation, histamine and leukotriene release.
42. Examples of soluble blood group antigens include, J antigen in cattle, R antigen in sheep, A antigen of pigs and DEA 7 antigen of dogs.
43. The red cell B system is also the major histocompatability system in the chicken.
44. HSP65 is major antigenic component of PPD.
45. PPD from *M. bovis* is more specific in cattle than *M. tuberculosis* giving less cross-reaction with *M. avium*.
46. All species mount a similar tuberculin reaction.
47. Horses appear to be unusually sensitive to tuberculin.
48. Allergic contact dermatitis belong to type I hypersensitivity.
49. The pathologic features of diseases caused by immune complexes reflect the site of immune complex deposi-

tion and are not determined by the cellular source of the antigen.

Match

50.

(1) Type I	-----	a. Cell mediated
(2) Type II	-----	b. Immune complex
(3) Type III	-----	c. IgE
(4) Type IV	----	d. ADCC

51. Define – Allergen

Allergen refers specifically to nonparasitic antigens capable of stimulating type I hypersensitive responses in allergic individuals.

Answers

1. Portier and Richet
2. Gell and Coombs.
3. IgE
4. atopy
5. P-K
6. IgG
7. Rhogam
8. macrophage
9. Serum sickness
10. a
11. d
12. b
13. e
14. d
15. d
16. b
17. False
18. False
19. True
20. False
21. False
22. True
23. False
24. True
25. True
26. True
27. True
28. True
29. False
30. False
31. False
32. False
33. True
34. True
35. True
36. True

37. True
38. True
39. True
40. True
41. True
42. True
43. True
44. True
45. True
46. False
47. True
48. False
49. True
50. 1.c,2.d,3.b,4.a

Chapter 21

Autoimmunity

Fill in the blanks

1. ____________are auto antibodies directed against the complement components C_2, C_4 especially C_3.

2. __________ is the prototype autoimmune disease mediated by blocking antibodies.

3. The immunodiagnostic test for autoimmune hemolytic anemias is _______ test.

4. Desensitization process used in immunotherapy of allergic diseases decreases specific IgE levels but increases____________ titrer.

Choose the best answer

5. The most important genes that influence naturally occurring autoimmune disease are

   (a) MHC (b) TCR

   (c) BCR (d) Complement

6. Rheumatoid factors are auto antibodies directed against which of the following isotype ?

   (a) IgG (b) IgM

   (c) IgE (d) IgA

7. SLE is most common in

   (a) young woman (b) old aged women

(c) Middle aged woman (d) Men

8. Which one of the following is not the mechanism for inducing autoimmunity ?

   (a) Release of sequestered antigen

   (b) Molecular mimicry

   (c) Polyclonal B cell activation

   (d) Tolerance

9. Which of the following can be used in treatment of autoimmune disease ?

   (a) Immunosuppressive drugs.

   (b) T cell vaccination

   (c) Peptide blockade of MHC molecule.

   (d) Monoclonal antibodies

   (e) all of the above

True or false

10. T cells can only be made tolerant to autoantigens if the T cells are first exposed to these antigens.
11. All autoimmune responses cause disease.
12. IK levels are nonspecific indicators of prevalence of infectious disease within an animal population.
13. Autoimmune diseases are much more common in women than in men.
14. Dogs, humans and chickens suffer from a naturally occurring autoimmune thyroiditis.
15. Diabetes mellitus is common in cattle.
16. Canine lupus affects males more than females.
17. IgG in rheumatoid arthritis patients is less glycosylated than normal IgG.

18. SLE produces elevated serum complement levels.
19. Unlike many other autoimmune diseases, 90% of the cases of ankylosing spondylitis are male.
20. Anti-TAC preferentially block auto reactive T cells.
21. T_H2 cells have been associated with development of autoimmunity.
22. A defect in the gene encoding Fas can reduce programmed cell death by apoptosis.
23. Serum sickness is the prototype for systemic immune complex-mediated disorders.
24. Immediate hypersensitivity reactions are dependent on the activation of T_H1 cells.
25. Mucosal mast cells have abundant histamine in their granules.
26. Athymic mice lack mucosal mast cells.
27. Prostacyclin causes smooth muscle relaxation.
28. Tryptase is specific to human mast cells.
29. IgG_4 is associated with atopic dermatitis in the dog.
30. In cattle, the major shock organ is lung.

Match

31.

1. Trypanosoma cruzi --- (a) Myelin basic
2. M protein by *Streptococci* ---- (b) Cardiac myosin
3. Epstein-Barr virus --- (c) Acetylcholine protein
4. Polio virus ---- (d) Nervous system receptor

Define

32. Molecular mimicry

Sharing of epitopes between an infectious agent or parasite and an autoantigen.

33. Epitope spreading

Autoimmune reactions initiated against oneself antigen may injure tissues, resulting in the release and alterations of other tissue antigens, activation of lymphocytes specific for these other antigens, and exacerbation of the disease. This phenomenon is called epitope spreading.

Answers

1. Immunoconglutinins
2. Myasthenia gravis
3. coombs
4. IgG
5. a
6. a
7. c
8. d
9. e
10. True
11. False
12. True
13. True
14. True
15. False
16. True
17. True
18. True
19. True
20. True
21. False
22. True
23. True
24. False
25. False
26. True
27. False
28. True
29. True
30. True
31. 1.d, 2.b, 3.a, 4.c

Chapter 22

Transplantation Immunology

Fill in the blanks

1. __________ reported the first systematic study of transplantation in 1908 in cats.
2. ________ showed lymphocytes are involved in graft rejection.
3. ________ test can be used to quantify the degree of class II MHC compatibility between potential donors and a recipient.
4. Major Histocompatability antigens are recognized directly by T_H and Tc cells, a phenomenon termed ________ .
5. Graft rejection occurs in two phases namely viz., ________ and ________ phase.
6. Cytokines primarily involved in graft rejection are _______, _______ and _______.
7. ________ , ________ and ________ are fungal metabolites with immunosuppressive properties.
8. CsA and FK506 exert their effect by binding to cytoplasmic proteins called ________ forming a complex that blocks the phosphatase activity of ________ .
9. Amino acid _______ is essential for T cell response.

10. Inhibition of liver allograft rejection appears to be due to the presence of enzyme __________ which destroys the aminoacid tryptophan.

11. __________ xenografts are those between clsoely releated species.

12. __________ xenografts are those between unrelated species, rejection is mediately largely by humoral mechanisms.

13. Humans and old-world monkeys lack the enzyme _______and has high levels of antibodies to the Galα1-3Gal epitope.

14. In allograft, ______ presentation involves recognition of an intact MHC molecule displayed by donor APCs and _____ presentation involved processing of donor MHC by recipient APCs.

Choose the best answer

15. T cell population involved in allograft rejection is

(a) $CD4^+$ (b) $CD8^+$

(c) both (d) None

16. For the purpose of organ grafting it can be assumed that there is only ________% chance of identity within MHC between siblings

(a) 12.5% (b) 25%

(c) 50% (d) 75%

17. Which statement is true about MLR when compared to microcytotoxicity assay ?

(a) Gives better indication of degree of T_H cell activation

(b) Takes several days

(c) Both are true

(d) None is true

18. Which cell generally serve as the major APC in graft ?

(a) Dendritic cells (b) Macrophages

(c) Both (d) None

19. Cells involved in alloantigen presentation are

(a) Passenger leucocytes (b) Langerhans cells

(c) Endothelial cells (d) All of the above

20. Effector mechanisms that participate in allograft rejection are,

(a) DTH (b) CTLs

(c) ADCC (d) All of the above

21. Cytokines produced by T $_{DTH}$ cells promote infiltration of which type of cell?

(a) Macrophages (b) Neutrophils

(c) CD8 cells (d) All of the above

22. Which of the following blood group antigen do not possess, carbohydrate side chain?

(a) ABO (b) Rh

(c) Lewis (d) None

23. Most commonly seen malignant tumors in allograft patients are,

(a) B cell lymphoma (b) Squamous cell carcinoma

(c) Both (d) Done

24. HLA matching before transplantation is usually done for

(a) Kidney (b) Liver

(c) Heart (d) None

25. Hyper acute rejection is mediated by,

(a) Pre-existing antibodies

(b) T_H cells

(c) Tc cells

(d) Macrophages

26. Xenografts are often rejected in .... manner

(a) Hyper acute (b) acute

(c) chronic (d) None

27. Which of the following is an example of a nondepleting antibody ?

(a) Anti CD3 (b) Anti IL-2R

(c) Anti CD4 (d) all of the above

28. Immune privileged sites include,

(a) Anterior chamber of eye,cornea

(b) Uterus

(c) Brain

(d) Cheek pouch of Syrian hamster

(e) All of above

29. Most frequently transplanted solid organ is

(a) Liver (b) Kidney

(c) Lung (d) Heart

30. To prevent GVHD

(a) Recipient is placed under immunosuppression

(b) Donar bone marrow treated with anti T cell sera

(c) both

(d) None

31. The potential problems associated with xenotransplantation is/are

(a) Hyper acute rejection (b) Xenozoonoses

(c) Both (d) None

32. When dogs are given MHC unmatched renal allografts, the grafts survive for about.

    (a) 24 h (b) 10 days

    (c) 40 days (d)2 months

33. Immune previleged sites accepts graft due to

    (a) Lack dendritic cells

    (b) lack MHC I & II

    (c) Blood-tissue barrier

    (d) Immuno-suppressive molecules

    (e) All of above

34. Pig organs are not successful in humans for grafting due to

    (a) Organ size mismatch

    (b) Xenozoonoses

    (c) Carbohydrate antigen

    (d) Lack of pig organs

35. Immunological destruction of fetus in pregnancy is prevented by,

    (a) lack of MHC Ia or II on preimplantation embryos

    (b) lack of MHC Ia or II on trophoblast

    (c) IFN-γ do not induce MHC expression in trophoblast cells.

    (d) Presence of HLA-G, HLG-E

    (e) All of above

True or false

36. Autografts and isografts are usually accepted owing to the genetic identity between graft and host.

37. In general skin grafts are rejected faster than other tissues such as kidney or heart.
38. Graft rejection attributes specificity and memory.
39. Second-set rejection is slower than first-set rejection.
40. Nude mice is capable of allograft rejection.
41. The blood group antigens are expressed only on RBCs.
42. Even when a fully HLA-compatible donor is not available, transplantation may be successful.
43. Intense proliferation of recipient T cells in MLR indicates good prognosis for graft survival
44. Matching or mismatching of the class I antigens has a lesser effect on graft survival unless there is mismatching of the class II antigens.
45. Kidney and bone marrow transplants may survive with greater mismatching.
46. Liver and heart transplants may survive with greater mismatching.
47. Successful transplantation even between HLA identical individuals requires some degree of immune suppression.
48. Minor histocompatability antigens are directly recognized by T_H and Tc cells.
49. Passenger leukocytes do not seem to play any role in skin grafts.
50. Passenger leukocytes are the only cells involved in immune stimulation.
51. The hallmark of graft rejection involving cell-mediated reactions is an influx of T cells and macrophages into the graft.
52. The IFNα, IFNβ, IFNγ, TNF-α and TNF-β all increase class I MHC expression.

53. Accelerated rejection is caused by antibodies that are produced immediately after transplantation.
54. Chronic rejection includes both humoral and cell mediated responses.
55. Both B cell and T cell proliferation is diminishing in the presence of Azathioprine.
56. CsA does not have any negative side effects.
57. FK506 and rapamycin are 10-100 times more potent as immune suppressants than CsA.
58. Exposure to anti-TAC after the graft specifically blocks proliferation of activated T cells.
59. Injection of anti CD3 monoclonal antibodies results in a rapid depletion of mature T cells from the circulation.
60. Lacking a co-stimulatory signal, antigen-activated T cells become anergic.
61. CD28 is expressed on both resting and activated T cells and binds B7 with a moderate affinity.
62. CTLA-4 is expressed at much lower levels and only on activated T cells but binds B7 with a 20 fold higher affinity.
63. There is no immunologic barrier to transplantation of cartilage or heart valves as they lack alloantigen.
64. Non-identical twins in cattle retained the ability to accept grafts from the genetically district sibling throughout their lives.
65. GVDH reaction is the major problem in liver and bone marrow transplants.
66. Complete T cell depletion from donor bone marrow increases the likelihood that the marrow will be rejected.

67. Liver appears to resist rejection by hyper acute antibody mediated mechanisms.
68. Second-set rejection is a manifestation of immunological memory.
69. Passenger leukocytes are host dendritic cells that migrate into grafted tissue and act as APCs.
70. All allografts between individuals with identical HLA haplotypes will be accepted.
71. In humans and pigs, MHC class II molecules are also expressed on the endothelium of renal arteries and glomeruli.
72. Skin grafts from male donors placed on histocompatible females are usually rejected, although the reverse is not the case due to H-Y molecule in males.
73. Blood group antigens mainly stimulate B cells.
74. Chronic allograft rejection is responsive to immunosuppressive therapy.
75. Eye and testes are unique in that they express very high levels of CD95L.
76. Concordant rejection is largely mediated by cellular reaction.
77. Pig organs trigger a severe discordant xenograft rejection response in human mediated by natural anti carbohydrate antibodies.
78. Seminal plasma is immunosuppressive.
79. Sperm exposed to seminal plasma is nonimmunogenic, even after washing.
80. In general, pregnancy is associated with strong skewing of mother's immune system in favor of Th1 response.
81. There is no NK cell in pregnant porcine uterus.

82. IFN ω in humans and IFNτ in ruminants stimulate lymphocyte proliferation.

83. As many as 2% an individual's T cells are capable of directly recognizing and responding to a single foreign MHC molecule.

84. Natural antibodies exist for Rh antigens.

Match

85.

1. Autograft : (a) Between species
2. Isograft : (b) Genetically different individuals of same species
3. Allograft : (c) Between genetically identical individuals
4. Xenograft : (d) Same individual

86.

1. Hyper acute rejection – a) few weeks
2. Acute rejection – b) months to years
3. Chronic rejection – c) Within 24 h

87.

1. Azathioprine – a) folic acid antagonist
2. Cyclophosphamide – b) alkylating agent
3. Methotrexate – c) mitotic inhibitor

Answers

1. Alexis carrel
2. Avrion Mitchison
3. MLR
4. alloreactivity
5. Sensitization, effector
6. IL-2, IFNγ and TNF-β
7. Cyclosporine A, FK506 and rapamycin

8. immunophilins, calcineurin
9. tryptophan
10. indolamine dioxygenase
11. Concordant
12. Discordant
13. α 1,3 galactosyltransferase
14. direct, indirect
15. c
16. b
17. c
18. a
19. d
20. d
21. a
22. c
23. c
24. a
25. a
26. a
27. c
28. e
29. b
30. c
31. c
32. b
33. e
34. c
35. e
36. True
37. True
38. False
39. False
40. False
41. False
42. True
43. False
44. True
45. False
46. True
47. True
48. False
49. True
50. True
51. True
52. True
53. True
54. True
55. True
56. False
57. True
58. True
59. True
60. True
61. True
62. True
63. True
64. True
65. True
66. True
67. True
68. True
69. True
70. False
71. True
72. True
73. True
74. True
75. True
76. True
77. True

78. True
79. True
80. False
81. False
82. False
83. True
84. False
85. 1.d,2.c,3.b,4.a
86. 1.c,2.a,3.b
87. 1.c,2.a,3.b

Chapter 23

Tumor immunology

Fill in the blanks

1. A tumor that is not capable of indefinite growth and does not invade or metastasis is __________. Whereas a tumor that continues to grow and becomes progressively invasive is ________.

2. Two well-studied oncofetal antigens are ______________ and __________.

Choose the best answer

3. Which of the following is not true about transformed cells ?

   (a) Decreased requirement for serum

   (b) Anchorage - dependent

   (c) indefinite growth

   (d) none of above

4. Marek's disease induces tumor of

   (a) T cell (b) B cell

   (c) NK cell (d) all of the above

5. NK cells are concentrated mainly in

   (a) bone marrow (b) thymus

   (c) secondary lymphoid organ (d) All of above

True or false

6. Majority of cancers of colon, breast, prostate and lung are carcinomas.
7. Leukemia tend to grow as tumor masses, whereas lymphomas proliferate as single cells.
8. Sarcomas arise from endodermal or ectodermal tissues.
9. Most RNA viruses replicate in the cytosol and do not induce malignant transformation.
10. Viral oncogenes possess introns.
11. Conversion of a proto-oncogene into an oncogene appears to accompany a change in the level of expression of a normal growth-controlling protein.
12. The single most frequent genetic abnormality in human cancer is mutation in p53.
13. Acute leukemias tend to arise in less mature cells, whereas chronic leukemias arise in mature cells.
14. Tumor-specific antigens are unique to tumor cells and do not occur on normal cells in the body.
15. Tumor associated antigens are unique to tumor cells.
16. Even when the same chemical carcinogen induces two separate tumors at different sites in the same animals, the tumor antigens are distinct.
17. Virally induced tumors express tumor antigens shared by all tumors induced by the same virus.
18. Majority of tumor antigens are unique to tumor cells.
19. The presence of oncofetal antigens is not diagnostic of tumors but rather serves to monitor tumor growth.
20. The recognition of tumor cells by NK cells is MHC restricted.

21. All three types of interferon have been shown to increase class I MHC expression on tumor cells.
22. LAK cell populations are typically >90% activated NK cells.
23. TILs require 100 fold more IL-2 for their activity than LAK cells do.
24. Hereditary retinoblastoma results from over expression of a cellular oncogene.
25. Viral integration into the cellular genome may convert a proto-oncogene into a transforming oncogene.
26. All oncogenic retroviruses carry viral oncogenes.
27. LAK cells are tumor specific.
28. The immune response against a virus-induced tumor protects against tumor induced by the same virus.
29. Multiple copies of cellular oncogenes are sometimes observed in cancer cells.
30. Nude mice are no more susceptible than normal mice to chemically induced or spontaneous tumors.
31. Many tumor antigens induce tolerance in a manner similar to normal self-antigens.
32. RAG knockout mice suffer from an increased incidence of spontaneous tumors of the intestinal epithelium whereas RAG/STAT-1 knockout mice develop mammary cancers.
33. NK cells are found in thymus.
34. Some NK cells express CD8.
35. Metastatic tumor cells often fail to express MHC I.
36. KIR molecules are the major NK cell receptors in cattle.
37. IL-3 cytokine prevents the death of cultured NK cells.

38. Bovine NK cells are found in highest concentration in the spleen and peripheral blood.

39. NK T cells assume a Th1 phenotype upon maturation and increase their secretion of IFN-γ.

40. Antibodies are effective in destroying the cells in solid cancers.

41. CD95 L is normally expressed on CTLs and NK cells.

42. Serum of a tumor bearing animal may cause the tumors of other animals to grow even faster.

43. Tumor cells usually become malignant in one step.

44. Blocking antibodies are non complement activating antitumor antibodies.

45. IL-2 is extremely toxic when administered alone.

46. Immune response to tumors exhibit the defining characteristics of adaptive immunity.

47. Virus-induced tumors are the most immunogenic tumors known.

48. Hepatotoxicity and vascular leak syndromes are common problems with immunotoxin therapy.

Define

49. Antigenic modulation

Certain tumor-specific antigens have been observed to disappear from the surface of tumor cells in the presence of serum antibody and then to reappear after the antibody is no longer present. This phenomenon is called "antigenic modulation".

50. Immune surveillance theory

This theory held that body constantly produces neoplastic cells but that in a healthy individual the immune system rapidly recognizes and eliminates these cells through cell-mediated mechanisms. The theory suggested that progressive cancer would result if the cancer cells somehow evaded recognition by T cells.

Answers

1. benign, malignant
2. alpha-fetoprotein and carcinoembryonic antigen
3. b
4. a
5. c
6. True
7. False
8. False
9. True
10. False
11. True
12. True
13. True
14. True
15. False
16. True
17. True
18. False
19. True
20. False
21. True
22. True
23. False
24. False
25. True
26. False
27. False
28. True
29. True
30. True
31. True
32. True
33. False
34. True
35. True
36. True
37. True
38. True
39. True
40. False
41. True
42. True
43. False
44. True
45. True
46. True
47. True
48. True

Chapter 24

Evolution of immune system

Choose the best answer

1. IgA class is found in

   (a) fish (b) amphibian

   (c) reptiles (d) birds

2. Limulus amoebocyte assay is used to estimate

   (a) endotoxin level (b) protein

   (c) carbohydrate (d) fat

3. Major defense mechanisms of invertebrates include

   (a) phagocytosis (b) Melanin formation

   (c) antimicrobial peptides (d) all of above

4. Which of the following complement system is present in invertebrates ?

   (a) classical (b) alternate

   (c) lectin pathway (d) both b and

True or false

5. Fish antibodies can't agglutinate antigens.

6. Urodeles generally lack a bone marrow.

7. IgX has χ heavy chain found in xenopus.

8. All reptile antibody responses appear to be T-dependent.

9. Birds possess lymph nodes.
10. Bursectomised birds can't reject skin grafts.
11. In avian blood, T cells constitute between 60% to 70% of the total lymphocyte population.
12. Bird lymphocytes originate in the yolk sac and migrate either to bursa or to thymus.
13. Principal immunoglobulin in chicken serum is IgY.
14. IgY of bird consists of two heavy chains called upsilon chain.
15. IgY can cause precipitation or agglutination only in the presence of high salt concentration.
16. IgY has long hinge region.
17. Chicken IgA has 3 heavy chain C domains whereas mammalian IgA has 4 domains.
18. Chicken genome has only one functional V gene and one J gene for both light and heavy chains.
19. In birds, rearrangement of immunoglobulin genes is an ongoing process.
20. Acquired immune mechanisms are found only in advanced vertebrates.
21. Invertebrates rely exclusively on physical barriers and innate immune defenses to exclude microbial invaders.
22. Invertebrates do not possess phagocytic activity.
23. Defensins are found not only in insects but also in mammals and plants.
24. Invertebrates can reject allografts and xenografts.
25. Fish lysozyme is much more broadly reactive than the mammalian enzyme.
26. Cartilaginous and bony fish possess all three complement pathways.

27. Cartilaginous and bony fish have bone marrow.
28. Pronephros of fish is a lymphoid organ analogous to mammalian bone marrow and lymph nodes.
29. IgG is the most ancient of immunoglobulin classes and is found in both bony and cartilaginous fish.
30. IgNAR consists of heavy and light chains.
31. CD3 of chicken contains only two dimers.
32. Only certain phases of antibody response are temperature - dependent.
33. Vertebrates generally respond to antigens faster and more intensively at higher temperatures.

Answers

1. d
2. a
3. d
4. d
5. False
6. True
7. True
8. True
9. False
10. False
11. True
12. True
13. False
14. True
15. True
16. False
17. False
18. True
19. False
20. True
21. True
22. False
23. True
24. True
25. True
26. True
27. False
28. True
29. False
30. False
31. True
32. True
33. False

Appendix

Nobel prize winners in the field of immunology

- First Nobel prize in medicine was awarded to Emil von Behring in 1901 for the work on antitoxins.
- Robert Koch - tuberculin (1905).
- Charles Richet - Anaphylaxis (1913).
- Jules Bordet - Complement (1919).
- Karl Landsteiner- Blood groups (1930).
- Ehrlich and Metchnikoff 1908.
- Burnet - 1960.
- Rodney Porter and Edelman - Structure of Antibody 1972.
- Rosalyn Yalow - Radioimmunoassay 1977.
- George Snell - MHC genes 1980.
- Baruj Benacerraf- Ir genes 1980.
- Niels Jerne, Georges Kohler, Cesar Milstein – Mab 1984.
- Sutsumu Tonegawa - Antibody gene rearrangement 1987.
- Donnall Thomas and Joseph Murray - Organ transplantation 1990.
- Emil Unanue - antigen processing by macrophages.
- Harold Varmus - Novel cellular oncogenes 1989.

- Jacques Miller - Roll of thymus.
- Prus Nossal - One cell - one antibody rule.
- Ali Isaacs and Liudermann - Interferon.
- Peter Doherty and Zon Kernagel - MHC restriction.
- William Coley - Tumor immunotherapy.
- Peter Medewar – Tolerance.
- Luc Montaigner – AIDS 1982.
- Bengt Samuelson- Inflammatory mediators.
- Robin Coombs - Incomplete antibodies.
- Bruce Click - Bursa of Fabricius.